CW00551347

Interpreting Dental Radiographs

Quintessentials of Dental Practice – 5
Imaging – 1

Interpreting Dental Radiographs

By
Keith Horner
John Rout
Vivian E Rushton

Editor-in-Chief: Nairn H F Wilson
Editor Imaging: Keith Horner

Quintessence Publishing Co. Ltd.

London, Berlin, Chicago, Copenhagen, Paris, Milan, Barcelona,
Istanbul, São Paulo, Tokyo, New Dehli, Moscow, Prague, Warsaw

British Library Cataloguing in Publication Data

Horner, K. (Keith), 1958 –
    Interpreting dental radiographs. – (The quintessentials of dental practice)
    1. Teeth – Radiography
    I. Title II. Rout, P. G. J. (Peter Graham John) III. Rushton,
    V. E. IV. Wilson, Nairn H. F.
    617.6'07572

    ISBN 1850970521

ISBN 1–85097–052–1

Foreword

What proportion of procedures in general dental practice includes the interpretation of radiographs? All but a small percentage. It therefore follows that practitioners of all ages should be skilled in interpreting dental x-rays. This very readable book – Volume 5 in the Quintessentials for General Dental Practitioners Series – has been written to help the hard-pressed practitioner maintain and enhance these skills.

A mine of clinically relevant information, generously illustrated with high-quality radiographic images, *Interpreting Dental Radiographs* provides an authoritative and comprehensive guide to reading x-ray images. With an emphasis on those radiographic appearances that most frequently challenge even the most experienced of practitioners, this book is an invaluable aid to improved diagnosis. Exposing patients to ionising radiation and obtaining good-quality x-rays is to no avail if the information included in the images cannot be accurately interpreted. All those who read or possibly only dip into this book will without doubt gain new insight and understanding of the information included in dental x-rays – an outcome which can only enhance diagnostic acumen and patient care. *Interpreting Dental Radiographs* is an excellent addition to the Quintessentials for General Dental Practitioners Series, filled from cover to cover with information for immediate chairside application.

Nairn Wilson
Editor-in-Chief

Preface

Radiography is an essential tool in dental practice and almost all patients will need a radiograph at some point during a course of treatment. Successful radiography requires well-maintained and safe equipment, careful film handling, accurate technique and controlled processing. Once a radiograph is produced it must be interpreted correctly. This book aims to provide a guide to successful radiological interpretation.

In preparing the book, we made an early decision to focus principally upon the more common radiological diagnostic tasks. While the choice of subjects making up the chapters is fairly predictable, the content was influenced heavily by the correspondence each of us has had with dentists in general practice over the years. General dental practitioners frequently send radiographs to us for an opinion, a service we are happy to provide. Time has informed us that certain conditions, anomalies and lesions recur as diagnostic problems and we have used this experience to help design the book.

Radiology is an expanding clinical discipline, with new technologies adding to the traditional armamentarium of x-ray set and film or cassette. However, in this book we make no apologies for sticking with the more traditional images that make up the overwhelming workload of the average dentist. In particular, we have decided to concentrate upon intraoral radiography, although there are some exceptions. In some places we refer to "image receptor", to acknowledge the increasing use of digital radiographic systems in dentistry.

Keith Horner
John Rout
Vivian E Rushton

Contents

Chapter 1
Basic Principles

Aim

The aims of this foundation chapter are threefold: first, to give an understanding of the nature of the radiographic image and the factors that govern its formation; second, to recognise the limitations of radiographs; finally, to describe a systematic approach to image interpretation.

Introduction

Our eyes constantly expose our brain to "images". Our binocular vision allows us to cope with three-dimensions while our colour vision helps to characterise the subtle variations of the objects around us. In contrast, radiographs seem to present a far simpler view on things: x-ray images are two-dimensional and consist of black, white and shades of grey. Interpretation of radiographic images, however, poses very different challenges from those presented by everyday vision. An understanding of these is essential to interpretation.

What Makes the Image?

Image formation begins with a pattern of x-rays hitting the image receptor (film, intensifying screen/film combination or digital receptor). This pattern is recorded, either chemically (film) or electronically (digital radiography), and displayed as a pattern of densities. The image you see is dictated principally by three factors:
- the nature of the radiation
- the nature of the objects lying between the x-ray source and the receptor
- the characteristics of the image receptor.

The Nature of the Radiation

X-ray energy and intensity are the important factors here.

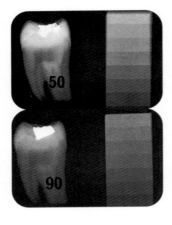

Fig 1-1 These images of a tooth and a small aluminium step wedge were produced at 50kV (top) and 90kV (bottom). The difference is subtle but the 50kV image shows greater contrast, seen most easily on the stepwedge.

X-ray energy

X-rays are high-energy, high frequency, short wavelength electromagnetic radiation. However, "x-rays" cover a band within the electromagnetic spectrum ranging from lower energy (lower frequency, longer wavelength) to higher energy (higher frequency, shorter wavelength). How the radiation that comes out of your x-ray set fits into this range of energies depends principally upon the kiloVoltage (kV). Most modern dental x-ray sets in the UK are in the 65 to 70kV band. Previously, many sets were manufactured to operate at 50kV. While the kV affects radiation dose, in this chapter we are concerned with the radiographic image. In this context, lower kV leads to high-contrast "black and white" images with few intermediate grey tones. Relatively higher kV produces images with more subtle variation in grey tones (longer grey scale) and lower overall contrast (Fig 1-1).

X-ray intensity

The greater the intensity of x-rays the more radiation hits the film. This produces a higher-density ("darker") image.

The Nature of the Object

The factors included in the "nature" of the objects are as follows.

Atomic number

This refers to the size of the atoms. High atomic number elements absorb x-radiation very effectively (Fig 1-2). Thus, materials like gold (atomic number = 79) absorb more radiation than calcium (atomic number = 20). High

Fig 1-2 The most striking example of the effect of atomic number upon x-ray absorption is seen with an everyday radiograph. This bitewing shows the enormous contrast difference between metallic restorations (high atomic number) and everything else. The gold crown is very radiopaque because of its very high atomic number, while the composite restorations in a number of teeth are comparatively radiolucent. The bone and teeth (moderately high atomic number elements) are, in turn, substantially more radiopaque than areas showing soft tissues (low atomic number elements).

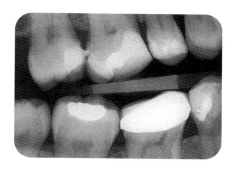

atomic number elements like barium (atomic number = 56) are added to some dental materials to make them radiopaque and thus help in making them visible on radiographs. In fact, the absorption of x-rays is proportional to the cube of the atomic number ("Z^3 effect"), making this an extremely potent influence on overall x-ray attenuation by materials.

Physical density
Atomic size is not the only factor of importance in x-ray attenuation. Physical density also plays a significant role. The most practical example of this is the contrast between air and soft tissues. While the mean atomic numbers of these are quite small, the relatively low density of air means that there is a very obvious contrast on radiographs at air/soft tissue boundaries (Fig 1-3).

Thickness and shape
Thicker objects absorb more x-rays than thinner ones of the same material.

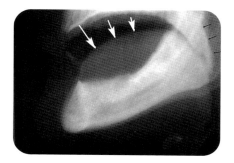

Fig 1-3 Air/soft tissue interfaces. Despite the fairly small difference in average atomic number between soft tissues and air, a visible contrast is present due to the large difference in density. The tongue outline is shown by white arrows, the soft palate posterior surface with black arrows.

Of course, in nature, objects are of variable thickness and usually have rounded margins. This means that in a two-dimensional radiograph the object will vary in its radiopacity according to its shape.

In practice, these three factors (atomic number, density and thickness) combine to govern the absorption of x-rays. However, the radiographic image depends upon the ability of the receptor (film, intensifying screen/film combination or digital receptor) to record and display the information in the attenuated x-ray beam.

The Characteristics of the Image Receptor

The important characteristics of the image receptor are:
- density
- contrast
- size of silver halide grains.

Density and contrast are partly governed by the characteristics of the objects in the x-ray beam (atomic number, physical density and thickness, as described above) but are also profoundly influenced by the radiographic process itself. In particular, image receptors all have individual "characteristic curves", that relate the density to the x-ray exposure. This relationship is only linear for some digital systems, all others being non-linear (Fig 1-4). The reasons for this, and the details of the curves for different image recep-

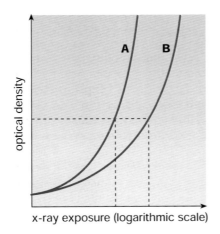

Fig 1-4 Characteristic curve for dental x-ray film(s). Optical density (vertical axis) indicates the "darkness" of the film. For the same density, film A requires less exposure than film B. Film A is, therefore, the faster film.

4

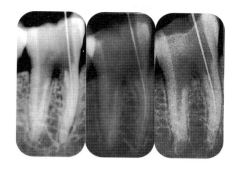

Fig 1-5 Three radiographs of the same tooth, taken using conventional dental film (right), an intensifying screen/film cassette combination (centre) and a digital intra-oral x-ray system (left). The difference in image sharpness is obvious, with conventional dental film being best. Indeed, at this magnification the grains of this fast emulsion (F-speed) dental film are visible.

tors, are not relevant to this book. The important point is that changing the image receptor (e.g. changing from one manufacturer of film to another) will have effects upon the character of the image you see, all other factors being equal.

The size of the silver halide grains in the emulsion has a strong influence upon the ability of a radiograph to differentiate between structures that lie close together (resolution). Resolution is objectively measured by radiographing test objects containing very fine metal wires of decreasing thickness and intervening distance. It can be expressed as the number of line pairs per millimetre (l.p. mm⁻¹). Dental intraoral film has very high resolution – around 20 l.p.mm⁻¹ – greater than the detail visible to the unaided human eye. This explains why magnification of intraoral (periapical, bitewing) radiographs not only increases image size but also improves the detail that can be perceived. Most intensifying screen/film cassette combinations, such as would be used for panoramic radiography, have a resolution of around 5 to 6 l.p. mm⁻¹, explaining why radiographs produced using cassettes can never reproduce detail as well as intraoral film. The resolution of digital receptors used for intraoral radiography has been estimated at between 6 and 15 l.p. mm⁻¹, depending on the system used. This, in part, may explain research findings that reveal that some intraoral digital systems are less effective at demonstrating fine root canal systems and fine endodontic files than conventional film. Three images of the same object on different image receptors that demonstrate resolution differences are shown in Fig 1-5. Using larger grain sizes is one way of increasing film speed. Thus, higher speed to reduce dose to patients involves a trade-off in terms of a reduction in sharpness of the image. Image sharpness is discussed in more detail below.

How "Accurate" is a Radiographic Image?

We tend to rely a lot on radiographs in dentistry. This reliance is based upon a trust that the image represents the truth accurately. In reality, no radiographic image can be a perfect representation of life. Some of the factors that should be considered are:
- magnification
- image sharpness
- spatial perspective
- temporal perspective.

Magnification

All conventional radiographic images are magnified. Radiographs are "shadow pictures" and the size of the shadow depends upon the relative relationship of x-ray source, object and image receptor.

$$\text{Magnification of the object} = \frac{\text{size of the image}}{\text{size of the object}}$$

But we can use simple geometry (Fig 1-6) to redefine magnification as:

x-ray source to film distance/x-ray source to object distance

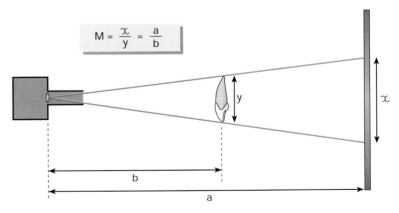

$$M = \frac{x}{y} = \frac{a}{b}$$

Fig 1-6 Magnification (M) can be defined as the size of the image divided by the size of the object. It is easier to measure in practice, however, by dividing the source to film distance by the source to object distance.

Thus, to produce an image with as little magnification as possible, we would choose an arrangement where the object was as close to the film as possible and where the x-ray source was far away from both. Many old dental x-ray machines used a very short x-ray source-to-skin distance (10cm). These gave relatively high magnifications compared to the modern machines using a 20cm or 30cm x-ray source-to-skin distance. Because magnification cannot be eliminated in conventional radiography we should use reference markers of known length when measuring distances, e.g. files in endodontic working length estimation.

In digital radiography, images are displayed on the computer monitor at various stated magnifications. However, it is important to remember that a "life-size" image (x 1 magnification) refers to the size of the object as recorded on the digital receptor surface, and will still have some magnification depending on the geometric relationship of x-ray source/object/receptor described above.

Image Sharpness

A radiographic image is always less "sharp" in its outline and its internal detail than the original object. In part, this is related to the fact that, inside the x-ray machine, the radiation derives from an area (the focal spot) rather than an infinitely small point (Fig 1-7). Thus, the "umbra" (= "shadow") of an object will be surrounded by a "penumbra", or peripheral blur. Clearly, the bigger the focal spot of the x-ray machine, the greater the blurring. Most dental x-ray sets have a focal spot about 1 mm in width. Focal-spot size tends to increase over years of use. Therefore, at least in theory, years of use will lead to a gradual reduction in image sharpness.

Penumbra size increases as the distance from focal spot to object decreases and that from object to image receptor increases, as shown in Fig 1-8. Thus,

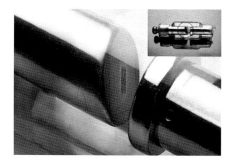

Fig 1-7 x-rays are produced in an x-ray tube (inset image). The main picture shows a close-up of the anode. The focal spot is visible as a small rectangular area on the anode surface.

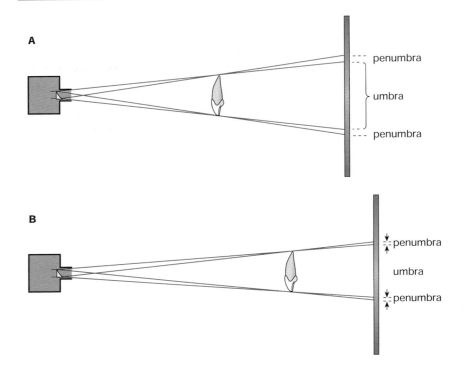

Fig 1-8 Penumbra, or peripheral blurring, is produced by the fact that x-rays are produced not from a point source but from an area (A). The size of the penumbra is reduced by moving the object closer to the film, or by increasing the distance from the source to the object and film (B).

for intraoral radiography the "ideal" situation is to have a very long distance from x-ray source to the patient, with the image receptor as close to the tooth as possible (exactly the same "ideal" as that for reducing magnification). With the paralleling technique for intraoral periapical radiography, the film has to be placed at a distance from the tooth and a longer focus-to-skin distance is needed compared to the old bisecting angle technique, where the film could be pressed closely to the tooth. This is why the paralleling technique is sometimes called the "long-cone" technique.

Sharpness is also influenced by the characteristics of the image receptor (as discussed above).

Spatial Perspective

On radiographs the three dimensions (height, width and depth) are converted to just two (height and width). Inevitably, therefore, the observed image depends upon perspective.

In the dental context, an appreciation of depth in an image is often gained by prior knowledge of normal anatomy. For example, we know that the incisive (nasopalatine) foramen lies to the palatal side of the upper central incisors. However, where anatomical knowledge is not helpful, three-dimensional appreciation can only be restored to radiography by viewing two radiographs with a differing perspective. At its simplest, this will involve taking two images at right angles (Fig 1-9). However, two images with only marginal differences in perspective allow interpretation of three dimensions by using the principle of parallax.

Principle of Parallax Localisation

- Take two radiographs of the same area with a perspective difference, usually a shift of beam angle of at least 20°.
- View the films in an orientation that matches this perspective shift.
- Pick a reference point/object of known position that is visible on both radiographs.
- Identify how the object of unknown position moves relative to the perspective shift.
- If the object seems to move in the **same** direction as the perspective shift, it is **lingual**/palatal to the reference object. If it moves in the **opposite** direction it is **buccal** in position. This is the "SLOB" rule.

A practical example of the use of parallax for localisation of an object is illustrated in Fig 1-10.

Perspective is a valuable tool for dentists, not least in uncovering information that is obscured by superimposition. For example, roots and root canals in multirooted teeth can be revealed by taking two periapical radiographs (Fig 1-11).

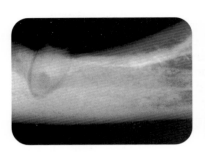
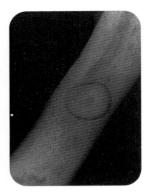

Fig 1-9 Example of retained root localisation using radiographs taken at right angles (periapical and true occlusal). The occlusal view (right) demonstrates that the mandibular canal passes lingually to the root.

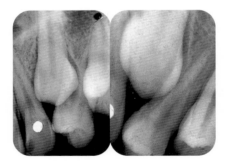

Fig 1-10 Example of parallax localisation of 23. Image 1 (on the left) was taken directly over the 23 region, while image 2 (on the right) was centred upon the premolar region. The 23 appears to have moved mesially relative to 22 and 24 in moving from image 1 to image 2, indicating that it is buccally located.

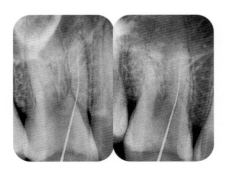

Fig 1-11 Changing relative position of upper molar roots on parallax. The image on the right is the orthogonal (90° to the arch) image, showing the mesiobuccal root superimposed upon the palatal root. The image on the left was taken with a 20° horizontal angulation (pointing mesially) and the mesiobuccal root has been projected clear of the other roots by parallax.

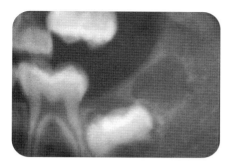

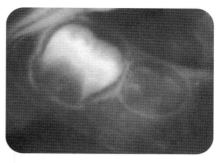

Fig 2-8 Crypt of 38, showing no calcification.

Fig 2-9 Earliest calcification in crypt of
38, showing just the cusps of the developing tooth. The 37 has complete crown
formation.

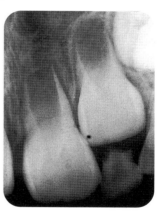

Fig 2-10 Developing roots of 21 and 22.

usually visible as a continuous, radiopaque, rounded "cap" over the "open"
apex (Fig 2-10).

Details of the normal development dates of the permanent dentition as seen
on radiographs are given in Table 2-1.

Alveolar Bone

Alveolar bone is predominantly trabecular in nature. The buccal and lingual
surfaces of the alveolar bone are covered in a thin layer of compact bone (cortex), but this is not visible radiographically on periapical radiographs. Compact bone is only visible in the form of the lamina dura of the tooth and some-

Table 2-1. **Normal development of the permanent dentition as seen on radiographs.**

	Tooth	Initial calcification	Crown complete	Eruption	Root(s) half complete	Root(s) complete
Maxilla	1	3-4 months	4 years	7-8 years	7 years	10 years
	2	10 months	4-5 years	8-9 years	7-8 years	10-11 years
	3	4 months	5-6 years	11-12 years	8 years	13-14 years
	4	2 years	6 years	10-11 years	9-10 years	12-13 years
	5	3 years	6-7 years	10-12 years	10 years	13-14 years
	6	birth	3 years	6-7 years	6 years	9-10 years
	7	3 years	7 years	12-13 years	11 years	15-16 years
	8	9 years	13-16 years	17-21 years	16 years	18-25 years
Mandible	1	2-4 months	4 years	6-7 years	6 years	8-9 years
	2	3-4 months	4 years	7-8 years	6-7 years	9-10 years
	3	4 months	4-5 years	9-10 years	7-8 years	12-14 years
	4	2 years	5-6 years	10-12 years	9 years	12-13 years
	5	3 years	6-7 years	11-12 years	10 years	13-14 years
	6	birth	3 years	6-7 years	6 years	9-10 years
	7	3 years	7-8 years	11-13 years	11 years	15-16 years
	8	9 years	12-16 years	17-21 years	16-18 years	18-25 years

Figures are average values and should be treated as a guide only. Eruption dates of up to two years of those shown would still be "normal". Generally, tooth development in females is in advance of males.

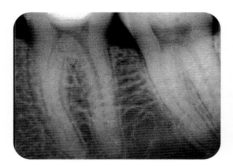

Fig 2-11 "Step ladder" trabeculation between roots of the lower molars.

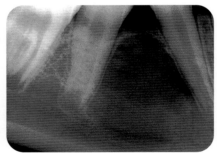

Fig 2-12 "Empty" trabecular pattern in the body of mandible. Note the intact lamina dura on the teeth.

times at the crest of the interdental bone. Trabecular pattern is highly individual. Indeed, it may sometimes be useful in forensic work for identification purposes. It is, therefore, difficult to make generalisations about "typical" features. However, maxillary bone usually has more numerous trabeculae than the mandible. The orientation of the trabeculae interdentally and interradicularly in the mandible frequently has a horizontal pattern that can be likened to the rungs of a stepladder (Fig 2-11). Nevertheless, in many cases the mandibular trabecular bone has a very open, almost featureless, radiolucent appearance (Fig 2-12). In these cases, the key feature of normality remains the continuity of the lamina dura around the teeth.

The Maxilla

Anterior region
This is the most anatomically complex region of the jaws. A number of key structures are visible on intraoral radiographs. The midline can be identified by a number of features. Superiorly, there is the inferior aspect of the nasal septum, with the nasal cavities on either side (Fig 2-13). At the base of the nasal septum there is a radiopaque, diamond-shaped structure: the anterior nasal spine (Fig 2-13). Running inferiorly from this, down to the alveolar crest, is the radiolucent midline suture (Fig 2-13). Overlying the suture and at a level corresponding to the apical or middle thirds of the roots of the central incisors is an area of radiolucency, the incisive (nasopalatine) foramen. This has notable variation in appearance, ranging from a single well-defined oval radiolucency to a more complicated arrangement of small radiolucencies (Fig 2-14). A more "classic" appearance is of a relatively indistinct radiolucency with thin radiopaque edges laterally, the latter resembling typewritten brackets (Fig 2-15). The incisive foramen is typically about 6 mm in width, but may normally be as much as 10 mm wide. If a periapical radiograph of an upper central incisor is taken, the image of the foramen may be moved by parallax to overlie the root and lead to interpretation as periapical inflammatory disease (Fig 2-16).

Other structures in the region of the anterior maxilla may intrude on periapical radiographs. The soft tissues of the (external) nose may be visible (Fig 2-17). These are visible because of the contrast with the surrounding air. Consequently the nostrils and intranasal airways are often distinct as radiolucent bands running vertically. In bisecting-angle technique periapical radiographs and the anterior occlusal projection it is sometimes possible to visualise the inferior conchae (turbinate bones) in the nasal cavities (Fig 2-17).

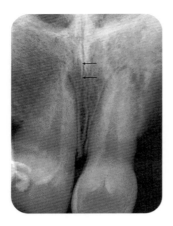

Fig 2-13 Anterior maxillary periapical showing the radiopaque "diamond" shape of the anterior nasal spine superiorly. The nasal septum runs upwards from this, with the radiolucent nasal cavities on either side. The midline suture (black arrows) runs downwards between the roots of the central incisors to the alveolar crest.

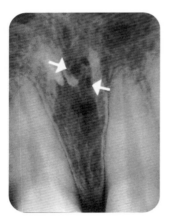

Fig 2-14 Multiple small radiolucencies form the incisive foramen in this patient.

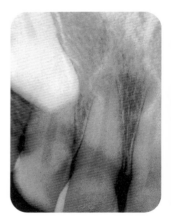

Fig 2-15 "Bracket" form of incisive foramen. This film was taken for 11, so the incisive foramen is moved by parallax slightly to the right side.

Canine/premolar region

The most prominent radiological features in this region are the anterior wall of the maxillary sinus and floor of the nasal cavity. These join in a characteristic way to form the "Y-line of Ennis" (Fig 2-18). Despite the name, this junction sometimes appears more akin to the letter "X" (Fig 2-19).

Canalis sinuosus, a prominent neurovascular channel, is sometimes visible

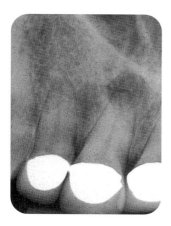

Fig 2-16 Incisive foramen moved by parallax over apex of the 11.

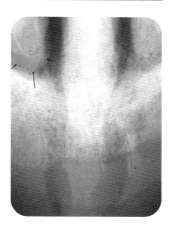

Fig 2-17 Soft tissues of external nose are clearly visible on this radiograph of an edentulous anterior maxilla. The inferior conchae are the rounded radiopacities in the nasal cavities (arrowed on the patient's right).

around the level of the lateral incisor or canine root apex (Fig 2-20) and should not be confused with a periapical inflammatory lesion.

The soft tissue image of the nasolabial fold, produced by the contrast between the thick cheek soft tissues and the thinner lips, passes obliquely across films in this region.

Molar region

The maxillary antrum dominates the bony anatomy in the molar region of the maxilla. Hypoplasia of the antrum, however, is a fairly common anomaly and leads to some patients' radiographs showing little or no evidence of an air space. The sinus floor has a thin cortical bone margin (a lamina dura). Where the roots of the teeth are related to the antrum, the lamina dura of the root and that of the antrum become one. Confusion in diagnosis sometimes arises because the radiolucent antrum is confused with a cystic lesion. The key factors in differentiation of antrum from cyst are that in a normal antrum:

• the antral floor is continuous and of uniform thickness

25

- normal dental lamina dura is (in health) present around related roots
- neurovascular channels are present in the antral wall (Fig 2-21).

These channels are not usually evident in pathological lesions such as cysts. While the antral floor runs smoothly across an upper molar periapical radiograph of many patients, in others septa may be present passing vertically from the floor (Fig 2-21), sometimes giving a loculated appearance to the antrum. The mucosal lining of the sinus is normally around 1 mm thick and (at this thickness) not radiologically visible.

Above the first or second molar, a radiopaque "U" is visible (Fig 2-22). This is the zygomatic process of the maxilla. In bisecting angle technique periapicals the downward x-ray beam casts this image over the roots of the teeth, leading to poor diagnosis. In contrast, paralleling technique radiography allows the image of the zygomatic process to be cast at or above the root apices (Fig 2-23). The inferior margin of the zygoma, leading towards the

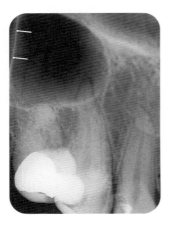

Fig 2-18 Y-line of Ennis. The rounded radiolucency is the anterior part of the maxillary antrum, into which the root apices of 13 and 14 project. Note the widened periapical periodontal ligament space on 23. At the distal edge of the film is a septum in the wall of the antrum (arrowed).

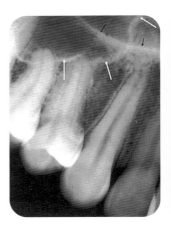

Fig 2-19 Here the radiopaque lines of the nasal floor (black arrows) and antral floor (white arrows) cross to form an "X" shape.

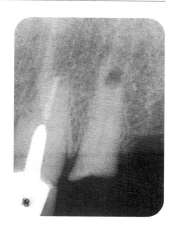

Fig 2-20 Canalis sinuosus overlying the root apex of this root. Note the faint outline of the canal running up from the radiolucency.

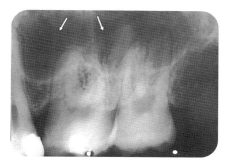

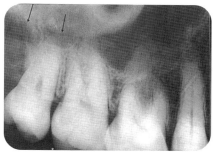

Fig 2-21 The neurovascular canal (arrowed) passes in a smooth curve overlying the image of the left maxillary antrum. The thin vertical radiopacity above 26 is a septum of bone.

Fig 2-22 Periapical radiograph of upper right teeth showing the "U"-shaped opacity of the zygomatic process of the maxilla (top of image) and the lower border of the zygoma passing posteriorly (arrowed).

zygomatic arch, appears as a band of opacity running posteriorly from the process.

Third molar region
Radiographs of upper third molars will demonstrate the maxillary tuberosity but may, if placed far enough posteriorly, show the pterygoid hamulus and the lower border of the lateral pterygoid plate. If periapical radiographs are taken using the bisecting angle technique, the mouth is open and the tip

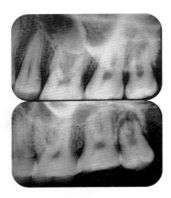

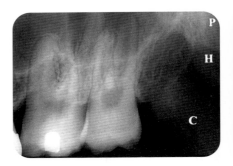

Fig 2-23 Periapicals of the upper molar region using the bisecting angle (top) and paralleling (bottom) techniques. The bisecting angle technique produces a distorted view of the molar roots and superimposition of the zygomatic process over the roots.

Fig 2-24 The pterygoid hamulus (H), lateral pterygoid plate (P) and coronoid process (C).

of the coronoid process will appear as a radiopacity on the inferodistal corner of the radiograph (Fig 2-24).

The Mandible

Anterior region

The midline of the mandible is marked by a radiopacity, the lingually placed genial tubercles. In the centre of this opacity a tiny radiolucency is usually seen, produced by the lingual foramen (Fig 2-25). This carries terminal neurovascular branches of the incisive canals. On occlusal radiographs the genial tubercles protrude prominently (Fig 2-26). To either side of the genial tubercles there are linear radiopaque bands called the mental ridges. These are simply due to the shape of the outer surface of the mandible and vary from patient to patient in their prominence (Fig 2-27).

Premolar region

The important anatomical structures in this region are the mandibular (inferior dental; inferior alveolar) canal and the mental foramen. The mental canal,

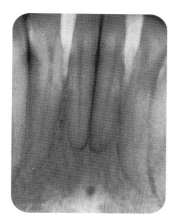

Fig 2-25 The small radiolucency below 31 and 41 is the lingual foramen. The relative radiopacity around and below this represents the genial tubercles.

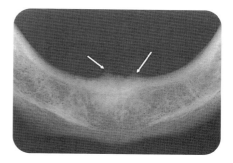

Fig 2-26 The genial tubercles (arrowed) viewed on a mandibular true occlusal radiograph.

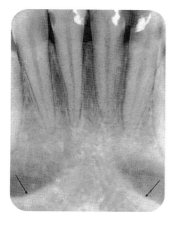

Fig 2-27 Mental ridges (arrowed) forming symmetrical radiopacities.

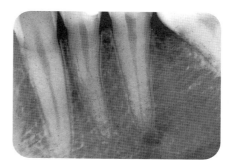

Fig 2-28 Mental foramen over apex of 35. Note the intact apical lamina dura on this tooth.

being the short branch of the mandibular canal leading to the foramen, passes upwards and posteriorly to reach the surface. The most common site for the foramen is approximately between the first and second premolar apices.

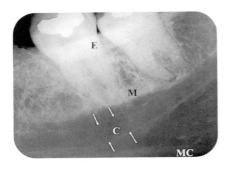

Fig 2-29 Molar periapical radiograph showing the external oblique ridge (E), mylohyoid line (M), mandibular canal (C; arrowed) and the inferior mandibular cortex (MC).

However, it frequently overlies the apex of a premolar (Fig 2-28). Its buccal location, however, means that it may appear anterior or posterior to this by parallax, depending on beam angulation. Its shape and prominence vary between patients and multiple foramina have been reported. While all dentists are aware of the mental foramen, it is sometimes mistaken for a periapical inflammatory lesion. Unless the tooth does indeed have a periapical lesion, careful examination of the film should reveal an intact periapical lamina dura. If confusion persists, parallax films will shift the foramen away from the root apex.

Molar region
The first molar region will, if a periapical film is placed deeply enough, show the mandibular canal running along the lower edge of the radiograph. One feature that occasionally causes diagnostic concern is a generalised radiolucency of the bone in this region (Fig 2-12). This is simply non-trabeculated marrow space.

The second/third molar region of the mandible is marked by a series of roughly parallel lines, running obliquely across periapical radiographs (Fig 2-29). Superiorly, the dense cortical bone of the external oblique ridge is always apparent. The next line is the mylohyoid line, the muscle attachment on the lingual surface of the mandible. This structure tends to be more apparent on bisecting angle rather than paralleling technique films. Below this, two parallel radiopaque lines are the walls of the mandibular canal. Inferior to the mylohyoid line the bone appears much more radiolucent. This is due to the depression of the submandibular fossa on the lingual aspect of the mandible. If the apices of teeth lie below the mylohyoid line, then the periapical periodontal ligament space will tend to be more radiolucent and give an impression of being widened that may lead to a false-positive diagnosis of pathology. Finally, at the lower border of the mandible, the cortical bone

Table 3-1. **Intervals between bitewing examinations based upon caries risk assessment. Caries risk should be reassessed at each visit. Intervals can be extended beyond 24 months in adults if there is continuing evidence of low caries risk.**

	Primary dentition	Permanent dentition
Low caries risk	12-18 months	24 months
Moderate caries risk	12 months	12 months
High caries risk	6 months	6 months

Monitoring Proximal Caries

A single bitewing radiograph is an image of a moment in time, providing no information on progression of caries. Demineralisation without cavitation may undergo remineralisation or progression and radiography offers the dentist an opportunity to monitor disease. In permanent teeth, it may take three to four years for caries to penetrate enamel. The rate of progression in dentine is less well studied. Progression rates vary from patient to patient and have a relationship to caries risk status.

Guidelines on frequency of bitewing radiography take caries risk into account. Current guidelines in the UK are shown in Table 3-1.

Monitoring of caries needs reproducible images if interpretation of any changes is going to be meaningful. Thus, the use of film holders and beam-aiming devices is essential, as are identical exposure factors to ensure consistent image contrast.

Occlusal caries

The primary method of occlusal caries diagnosis is careful clinical inspection. The diagnostic usefulness of radiography is limited because the occlusal caries is superimposed by the full buccolingual width of the tooth. Thus, in the early lesion there is substantial overlying sound enamel and dentine and enamel-only occlusal caries is not reliably identifiable radiographically. Furthermore, the extent of occlusal caries in dentine is underestimated. Radiological evidence of dentinal occlusal caries is strongly associated with heavily infected dentine. Despite these facts, studies have shown that bitewing radiography offers a useful diagnostic yield over clinical examination alone.

Occlusal caries appears as a spot or line of increased radiolucency immediately underneath the ADJ (Fig 3-8). As the caries extends, it forms a semicircular radiolucency with its flat surface against the ADJ (Fig 3-9). However, even at this stage there may be no perceptible enamel defect. In some teeth with dentinal occlusal caries, a band of increased radiopacity may be seen between the lesion and the pulp (Fig 3-10). This is due to increased calcification within the deeper dentine, presumably a host response to the advancing lesion. Enamel radiolucency is usually only seen when the den-

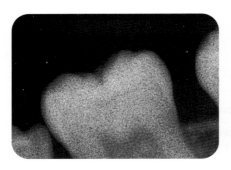

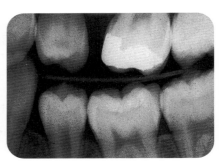

Fig 3-8 In 36, there is a slight increase in radiolucency below the CEJ, indicating early caries in dentine.

Fig 3-9 Deeper occlusal lesions. On this bitewing film lesions extending well into dentine are visible on 24, 37 and 36. The enamel, however, is radiologically intact.

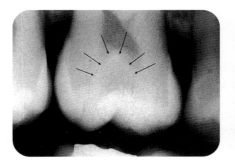

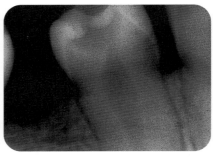

Fig 3-10 Increased opacity below occlusal lesion. In the 16 the edge of the deep occlusal caries lesion is marked by a subtle increase in radiopacity (arrowed).

Fig 3-11 In this very deep occlusal lesion, a small enamel radiolucency is visible.

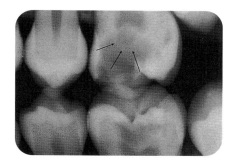

Fig 3-12 This film shows very deep caries in upper and lower first molars. In the upper molar there is a thin radiopaque layer of secondary dentine overlying the pulp (arrowed).

tine caries is advanced (Fig 3-11). Secondary dentine may reduce pulp size in relation to the advancing caries lesion, or at least maintain a barrier around the pulp (Fig 3-12).

Factors Affecting Radiological Interpretation of Occlusal Caries

As with proximal caries diagnosis, we rely on our ability to recognise the occlusal lesion by its contrast. Thus, the same factors of film type, exposure, kV and processing all have influences on perceptibility. A low contrast radiograph, whatever its cause, will reduce your ability to see an occlusal lesion if present, increasing the proportion of false-negative diagnoses.

A further confounding factor is an optical illusion: the "Mach band". Where the eye encounters a sudden difference in density (a "light/dark" boundary), such as is seen at the ADJ, the perception is that there is a thin dark band on the lighter side of the junction. Interpretation of this phenomenon as caries will result in an increase in false-positive diagnoses.

Buccal or lingual caries may coincidentally lie directly over the ADJ and mimic occlusal caries. Such lesions are generally more localised and have sharper margins than occlusal caries.

The final problem is, as might be expected, observer variability. This has already been discussed above for proximal caries and the importance of good viewing conditions in improving observer performance must be repeated.

Buccal/lingual caries
These lesions, occurring in smooth surface pits and fissures or at the cervical margin, are not well demonstrated by radiography. Empirically it is easy to accept that this is due to superimposition of the lesion on the full thick-

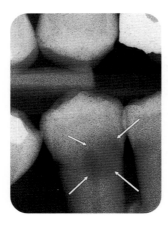

Fig 3-13 Smooth-surface (buccal) caries on 45 appears as an ovoid radiolucency, but would have been very obvious clinically. Smaller lesions may have no obvious radiological signs.

ness of the tooth. If they are visible they appear as round/ovoid well-demarcated radiolucencies (Fig 3-13). Depending on the site of the radiolucency, they can be misinterpreted as occlusal or proximal caries. Clinical examination is the key to diagnosis, with radiology offering little information useful to management.

Root Surface (Cemental) Caries

Root surface caries can occur at any point around the tooth immediately below the amelocemental junction. However, it is most often encountered on radiographs proximally. Lesions are radiolucencies on the root surface (Fig 3-14). They are usually shallow, although occasionally a "notched" appearance of the root surface is seen.

The main confounding factor in radiological diagnosis is cervical burnout. This is a phenomenon that relates to the additive effect of the curved shape of the mesial/distal root surface and the absence of overlying bone. As described in Chapter 1, the relatively thinner periphery of a cylindrical object leads to relative radiolucency. While most teeth do not have a perfectly cylindrical cross-section, varying degrees of curvature of the mesial and distal surfaces mean that this effect occurs on bitewing radiographs (Fig 3-15). Furthermore, where there is periodontal bone loss, the cervical portion of the tooth lacks overlying bone and appears more radiolucent than the root lying below the bone level. The cumulative effect is cervical burnout (Fig 3-16). Differentiation from root surface caries requires careful viewing with magnification. With caries there will be a saucerised defect in the root surface,

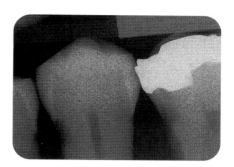

Fig 3-14 Root-surface caries in 34 distal, 35 mesial and 36 mesial. The lesions lie just below the CEJ.

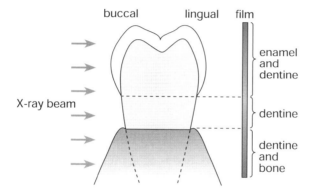

Fig 3-15 Cervical burnout. The gap between the CEJ and the alveolar bone crest only contains dentine. Thus there is less material in the cervical region to absorb x-rays, leading to a darker band across the radiographic image of the tooth. The rounded cross-section of most tooth roots accentuates this phenomenon peripherally, as can be seen in Fig 3-16.

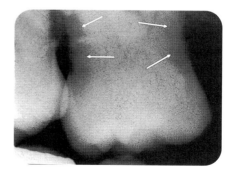

Fig 3-16 Cervical burnout. The mesial and distal surfaces of 16 have marked bands of burnout, which end abruptly at the alveolar bone margin.

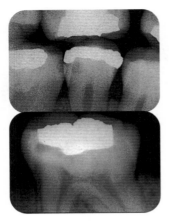

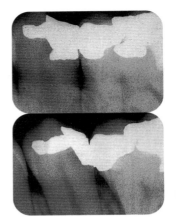

Fig 3-17 Secondary caries in 45 distally (top film) and occlusally in 36 (bottom film).

Fig 3-18 In the top image, there is only a suggestion of secondary caries below the distal part of the amalgam on 35. On the lower film, taken at the same examination, the recurrent caries is more obvious.

while with "burnout" the surface will be intact. Furthermore, cervical burnout will extend to the crestal bone level.

Secondary (recurrent) caries

Secondary caries is a common clinical problem. Radiology complements clinical examination by demonstrating lesions occlusally, distally and mesially. Recurrent caries is identified by its greater radiolucency as compared with adjacent dentine and/or by its greater contrast with adjacent radiopaque restorative materials (Fig 3-17). Radiopaque filling materials will, however, hide caries if the perspective is unfavourable (Fig 3-18).

The identification of secondary caries is hampered by the presence of radiolucent restorative and base materials.

Diagnostic validity of radiology in caries diagnosis

As described above, radiology lacks accuracy in the diagnosis of dental caries, although accuracies vary according to the type of caries, the depth of lesions and image quality. As dentists using radiographs on a daily basis, it is easy to

Table 3-2. **Diagnostic performance of radiography for the detection of caries.**

		Mean sensitivity	**Mean specificity**
Occlusal surfaces	dentinal	53	83
	enamel	30	76
	any	39	91
Proximal surfaces	cavitated	66	95
	dentinal	38	95
	enamel	41	78
	any	50	87

forget the limitations of radiographs for caries diagnosis, so it is useful to consider the diagnostic validity, as illustrated by sensitivity and specificity.

Sensitivity indicates the ability of the diagnostic method to identify lesions by ascribing a figure that states the proportion of lesions (%) that would be identified by the method ("true positive" fraction). Specificity is the proportion of healthy sites that would be correctly identified by the diagnostic method ("true negative" fraction). The perfect diagnostic system would have 100% sensitivity and 100% specificity. Sensitivities less than 100% indicate that there will be a proportion of undetected lesions of caries (false-negative diagnoses), while specificities less than 100% indicate that there would be a proportion of healthy surfaces misdiagnosed as carious (false-positive diagnoses). It is only by understanding these terms that you can quantify the diagnostic validity of different imaging techniques.

Bader and colleagues carried out a systematic review of dental caries diagnostic methods in 2001. Table 3-2 gives the mean sensitivities and specificities of radiography in caries diagnosis obtained by their review. It should be noted that the figures quoted represent the averages of studies and conceal fairly wide ranges, reflecting variable methodologies. We can, however, make some general points:
- specificity is invariably better than sensitivity
- sensitivity is better for more advanced carious lesions
- where all lesion depths are included, radiography identifies about half of proximal lesions.

- where all lesion depths are included, radiography identifies a minority of occlusal lesions.

It is worth contrasting these results with alternative diagnostic techniques. Visual examination of occlusal surfaces had a mean sensitivity of 59% and a mean specificity of 72% (any depth of lesion), while for electrical conductance methods the figures were 73% and 87% respectively.

The important point to recognise from the valuable review by Bader and colleagues is that radiography is not the "gold standard" for caries diagnosis and that it remains only a tool (albeit a valuable one) to help in managing patients.

Further Reading

Bader JD, Shugars DA, Bonito AJ. Systematic reviews of selected dental caries diagnostic and management methods. J Dent Educ 2001;65:960-968.

Gratt BM, White SC, Pharoah MJ. Dental caries. In: White SC, Pharoah MJ (Eds.) Oral Radiology. Principles and Interpretation. 4th ed. St Louis: Mosby, 2000.

Grondahl H-G. Radiologic diagnosis in caries management. In: Thylstrup A, Fejerskov O (Eds.) Textbook of Clinical Cariology. 2nd ed. Copenhagen: Munksgaard, 1994.

Langland OE, Langlais RP. Principles of Dental Imaging. 2nd ed. Philadelphia: Lippincott Williams and Wilkins, 1997: 395-411.

Whaites E. Essentials of Dental Radiography and Radiology. 3rd ed. Edinburgh: Churchill Livingstone, 2002: 217-227.

Chapter 4
Radiology of the Periodontal Tissues

Aim

To give a concise summary of how to image the periodontal tissues and to provide a comprehensive description of the radiological signs that must be identified for diagnosis of periodontal diseases.

Introduction

The primary diagnostic methods in the assessment of the periodontal tissues are history and clinical examination. Radiology thus serves as an adjunct to clinical assessment. Its principal functions are shown in Table 4-1. As discussed in Chapter 1, any radiograph is a "snapshot" in time; it only serves to provide evidence of the effects of past periodontal disease and does not give meaningful information about current disease activity.

Radiography of periodontal bone is surprisingly challenging. The three-dimensional shape of the bony supporting tissues of teeth is represented by a two-dimensional image. Thus, localised defects may be masked by superimposed bone. Where irregular defects are recognised, radiography alone cannot portray the three-dimensional shape.

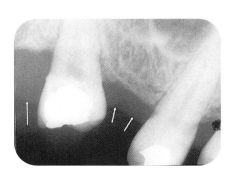

Fig 4-1 Radiograph of 17 and 15 showing gingival outline (arrowed).

Periodontal Disease Classification

This chapter deals with the general principles of interpretation of the periodontal tissues on radiographs. The gingival diseases are not included for the simple reason that they rarely have any radiological manifestations. Occasionally gingival hypertrophy may be visible radiographically and the thickness of gingivae assessed, particularly where there is a gap between teeth (Fig 4-1). However, as a generalisation, it is reasonable to say that radiology only serves a role in the management of the periodontal diseases. These diseases can be summarised as:

- plaque-induced periodontal diseases
    - aggressive periodontitis
        - *localised*
        - *generalised*
        - *recurrent*
    - chronic periodontitis
        - *localised* (< 30% sites)
        - *generalised* (> 30% sites)
        - *recurrent*
        - *refractory periodontitis*
- systemic diseases affecting periodontal tissues (e.g. pre-pubertal diseases such as hypophosphatasia, Papillon-Lefèvre syndrome).
- necrotising periodontitis
- lateral periodontal abscess
- periodontal-endodontic lesions.

All of these share the common feature of bone loss; their differences are in disease pattern and extent, age of onset, speed of progression and management. Details of these specific types of periodontal diseases can be found in textbooks of periodontology. Our role here is to highlight the job of interpreting the common radiological features.

Choice of Radiographs

In 1998, the Faculty of General Dental Practitioners' publication "Selection Criteria for Dental Radiography" established guidelines for radiography of periodontal diseases. While the strategy of the panel producing these guidelines was to assume an evidence-based approach, they emphasised that there was a paucity of good evidence to produce them. A revision of these guidelines has recently been carried out and the new guidelines are shown in Table 4-2.

Table 4-1. **The role of radiographs in assessment of the periodontal tissues.**

Identification of bone loss	present or absent?
Characterisation of bone loss	localised generalised horizontal pattern vertical defects furcation involvement apical disease bone density/quality loss of lamina dura widening of periodontal membrane space
Quantification of bone loss	absolute measurement ratio of CEJ to alveolar crest / CEJ to apex (approximation of % bone loss) bone loss over time
Identifying local aggravating factors	calculus poorly contoured restorations tilted teeth caries
Other associated features	evidence of occlusal trauma bone sclerosis as a response to disease maxillary sinus changes root resorption hypercementosis

The guidelines represent a pragmatic approach suitable for the general dental practitioner and are based upon the foundation of good quality posterior bitewing radiographs. For a dentate patient, bitewing radiographs should be taken at the first visit for caries diagnosis and repeated at appropriate intervals (see Chapter 3). These radiographs demonstrate the periodontal bone in the posterior regions, doing so using an optimal geometry. Thus, for patients with generalised regular bone loss no other radiographs may be needed. Vertical bitewing film holders are available commercially (Fig 4-2) for patients with clinical attachment loss greater than 6 mm. Of course, for many patients you will need to take two films for each side to cover all the posterior teeth using the vertical technique (Fig 4-3).

Table 4-2. **Guidelines (referral criteria) for radiography for periodontal disease.**

Clinical findings	Radiographs
Uniform pocketing < 6 mm and little or no recession	Horizontal posterior bitewings.
Uniform pocketing 6 mm or greater	Vertical posterior bitewings, supplemented by periapical radiographs using the parallel ing technique at sites where alveolar bone image is not included.
Irregular pocketing	Bitewing radiographs (horizontal or vertical depending on pocket depth), supplemented if necessary by periapical radiographs taken using the paralleling technique.

Based upon a history and the clinical examination, the category of 6 mm or greater is equivalent to a basic periodontal examination (BPE) sextant score of Code 4 (assuming no recession). However, remember that the BPE does not assess recession and therefore the GDP cannot rely on the BPE to record attachment loss: a 5 mm pocket adjacent to 4 mm recession is 9 mm attachment loss.

A dental panoramic radiograph (DPR) of optimal quality may offer a dose advantage over large numbers of intraoral radiographs and may be considered as an alternative if available. This may be the case when there are concurrent problems for which radiography is indicated – for example, symptomatic third molars, multiple existing crowns/heavily restored teeth and/or multiple endodontically treated teeth in a patient new to a practice. However, in view of the limitations in fine detail on DPRs, supplementary intraoral radiographs may be necessary for selected sites.

A traditional method of assessing the periodontal bone is the full-mouth periapical survey. This undoubtedly provides comprehensive coverage and allows calculation of residual bone support that facilitates prognostic decision-making. The full mouth survey requires many individual radiographs, however, adding to the radiation dose. Where periapical radiographs are taken, it is essential to use the paralleling technique. With the bisecting angle technique, particularly in the upper jaw, the angulation of the x-ray beam will project the buccal plate of bone coronally, masking periodontal bone loss (Fig 4-4).

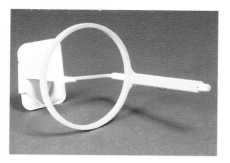

Fig 4-2 Vertical bitewing holder.

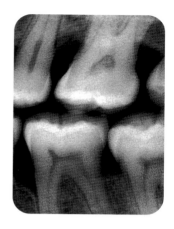

Fig 4-3 Vertical bitewing radiograph.

Fig 4-4 On the left is part of a bisecting angle technique radiograph, while on the right is part of a paralleling technique radiograph of the same patient showing less apparent bone loss using the bisecting angle technique due to the beam angulation.

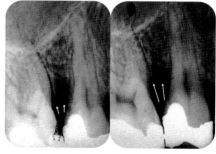

Dental panoramic radiographs (DPRs) are widely used for periodontal bone assessment. If you use panoramic radiography, then you should do so only with an understanding of its deficiencies. Image quality in the anterior regions may be poor due to the superimposition of the cervical spine. Overlap of teeth, as is often seen in the canine/premolar regions of even good quality DPRs, may make some sites unmeasurable. DPRs perform best for demonstration of periodontal bone in the mandibular premolar and molar regions. One study found that small areas of bone destruction were detected four times as frequently by intraoral radiography than by panoramic radiography. Other studies show conflicting evidence about the accuracy of DPRs, some suggesting an underestimation and others an overestimation of bone loss. Empirically, though, we can accept that the poorer image sharpness and the greater risk of "burnout" of the image with DPRs will lead to inaccuracies in assessing bone loss.

51

The "take home message" about radiographic selection is that bitewing radiographs offer information about caries *and* periodontal bone, and that the latter is shown on bitewings with the best image geometry achievable with simple radiographs. For more advanced periodontal disease, however, selective periapical views provide the only means of accurately assessing residual bone support.

Interpreting Periodontal Bone on Radiographs

The primary function of radiographs in the assessment of periodontal bone is to portray bone loss. Therefore there is a requirement to know the normal position of the crest of the periodontal bone. This level is between 0.5 and 1.9 mm below the CEJ (Fig 4-5). Other studies have defined thresholds for bone loss at a distance of up to 3mm.

Casual viewing of radiographs can lead to misinterpretation. We tend to assume that a normal periodontal bone level will be "horizontal" and even. However, where adjacent CEJs are not coincident in height, the periodontal bone will appear irregular and may give an impression of vertical bone defects (Fig 4-6).

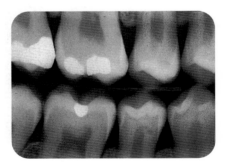

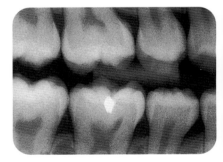

Fig 4-5 Normal periodontal bone levels on a bitewing radiograph.

Fig 4-6 Normal periodontal bone levels with an apparently irregular pattern (e.g. 16 mesially, 45 mesially). Note that the bone level mirrors the irregularity of the alignment of the adjacent cemento-enamel junctions. Small deposits of calculus are visible as "spurs" interproximally on the lower teeth and as a plaque mesially on 16.

Bone Loss

Having established what is normal, it is important to know the radiological signs of early bone loss. These are:
- "blunting" of the alveolar crest with blurring of the margin
- loss of the sharp angle between the lamina dura and alveolar crest.

These are very subtle changes that are far more difficult to diagnose reproducibly than to define theoretically. Furthermore, they are impossible to identify on the buccal/lingual tooth surfaces. This emphasises the overriding importance of good clinical examination rather than reliance upon radiology. If you are looking for these early signs of disease, then the use of ideal viewing conditions (Chapter 1) is paramount.

For the task of assessing bone loss, your eye should identify the CEJ and pass down the root surface until the lamina dura is reached (Fig 4-7). The degree of bone loss can thus be assessed on each visible mesial and distal tooth sur-

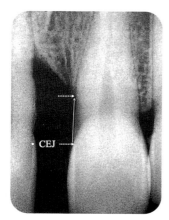

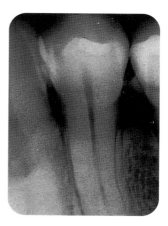

Fig 4-7 Magnified image of a tooth showing the method of assessing bone loss. Identify the cemento-enamel junction (CEJ) and follow the edge of the root downwards until the lamina dura is encountered. This distance, minus the normal 1.5-2 mm "gap" between CEJ and bone, equals the bone loss.

Fig 4-8 "Cervical burn-out". This film shows the "darkening" of the root between the cemento-enamel junction (CEJ) and the alveolar bone crest.

face, after taking into account the normal gap of approximately 2 mm. Bone loss can be classified as "mild" (1-2 mm), "moderate" (3-4 mm) or severe (> 5mm), although different experts have used these terms more subjectively. The bone level is far less easy to identify where it overlies the tooth and is complicated by superimposition of buccal and lingual crestal bone.

Of course, absolute measurement of bone loss in millimetres may not have the same clinical consequences for all patients. Root length varies from tooth to tooth and to a limited degree from patient to patient, so the concept of considering bone loss in terms of "crown:root ratio" can be used. This is the ratio of the tooth length beyond the level of bone to that supported by the bone. Alternatively, bone level may be expressed as a percentage of root length (CEJ to apex).

In mild bone loss, the increasing gap between the CEJ and the bone crest may produce a band of cervical burnout across the tooth (Fig 4-8). This becomes a wider band where bone loss is greater.

Furcation bone loss

As mild bone loss progresses to moderate bone loss, its identification becomes easier. A key sign to identify is the involvement of the furcation of a multi-rooted tooth (Fig 4-9). This is recognised in two ways:

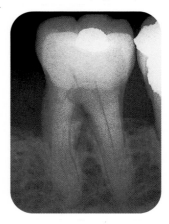

Fig 4-9 Furcation bone loss in 36.

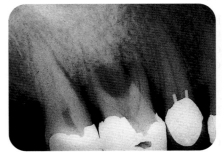

Fig 4-10 Furcation bone loss in 16. The palatal root tends to obscure the furcation, but careful examination shows the additional radiolucency of the root associated with loss of bone.

Hypercementosis

As with resorption, a direct causal relationship with periodontal diseases is not proven, but hypercementosis is seen occasionally on teeth with bone loss. It may be a response to inflammation or to the increased occlusal loading on a tooth with attachment loss. Hypercementosis appears as a thickening of the root with a normal surrounding periodontal ligament and lamina dura (Fig 4-17).

Aggressive Periodontitis

Aggressive periodontitis (previously known as early-onset periodontitis) may be localised or generalised. Localised aggressive periodontitis (still widely called "juvenile periodontitis") has a circumpubertal onset and is localised to first permanent molar and incisor teeth. Interproximal attachment loss is present at two or more teeth and involves no more than two non-first molar or incisor teeth. The precise age group of the patient and this characteristic distribution of affected sites (Fig 4-18) contribute to diagnosis. In contrast, generalised aggressive periodontitis has a broader age distribution, usually (but not exclusively) affecting patients < 30 years of age. There is generalised interproximal attachment loss affecting at least three permanent teeth that are not first molars or incisors.

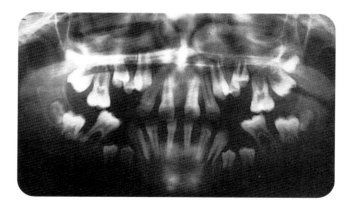

Fig 4-18 Aggressive periodontitis in a 10-year-old boy. There is extensive periodontal bone loss on the first molars and incisors. The anterior teeth are also spaced due to the degree of bone loss and drifting.

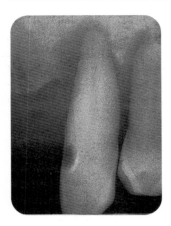

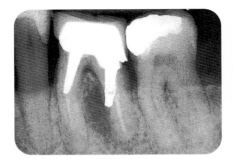

Fig 4-19 Lateral periodontal abscess on 43. The radiological appearance is of very advanced periodontal bone loss.

Fig 4-20 "Perio/endo" lesion of 36. There is periodontal bone loss affecting all the teeth, with some sign of furcation involvement of 36. The post in the distal root perforates into the furcation bone and is associated with inflammatory bone loss. The combined periodontal and endodontic problem led to treatment by resection of the distal root.

Lateral Periodontal Abscess

This is a rapidly developing infection developing in a deep pocket and leads to bone destruction that may be extensive. The primary diagnosis is clinical. The rapid development and destructive nature of the abscess, however, means that radiologically the principal feature is bone destruction (rarefying osteitis), with loss of lamina dura of the affected tooth that may extend periapically (Fig 4-19).

Periodontal/Endodontic Lesion

This entity is an incompletely understood phenomenon that may present clinically in a variety of ways. It refers to teeth (typically molars) that have concurrent clinical and radiological signs of disease of periodontal and pulpal origin. "Perio-endo" lesions may develop from an initial periodontal or endodontic lesion. Alternatively, it is argued that true "combined" lesions may develop. It certainly seems reasonable to argue that inflammation of pulpal origin may develop in periodontal defects via accessory pulp canals and that pulpal infection may drain via the periodontal ligament.

The typical radiological picture is of a heavily restored molar with evidence of periapical (or lateral) inflammation of pulpal origin and furcation radiolucency (Fig 4-20). A connection between the furcation lesion and the gingival margin may be identifiable clinically but is often not visible radiographically.

Further Reading

Hirschmann PN. Radiographic interpretation of chronic periodontitis. Int Dent J 1987;37:3-7.

Langland OE, Langlais RP. Principles of Dental Imaging. 2nd ed. Philadelphia: Lippincott Williams and Wilkins, 1997: 357-374.

Tugnait A, Clerehugh V, Hirschmann PN. The usefulness of radiographs in diagnosis and management of periodontal diseases: a review. J Dent 2000;28:219-226.

White SC, Pharoah MJ. Periodontal diseases. In: White SC, Pharoah MJ (Eds.) Oral Radiology. Principles and Interpretation. 4th ed. St Louis: Mosby, 2000: 290-302.

Chapter 5
Periapical and Bone Inflammation

Aim

The aim of this chapter is to provide the practitioner with an understanding of the radiology of common inflammatory conditions affecting the periapical regions and bone.

Introduction

Inflammation is the most frequent cause of altered radiological appearances in the periapical region. Demineralisation of between 30% and 60% of hard tissue is necessary before radiological signs of pathosis become apparent. This process can take up to ten days, hence the delay between the onset of clinical signs and symptoms and their radiographic appearance.

Choice of Radiographs

The traditional method of assessing the status of the periapical region of a tooth is by intraoral periapical radiography. The paralleling technique is preferable to the bisecting angle technique as the latter can result in geometric inaccuracies that may distort or obscure apical pathology (Fig 5-1).

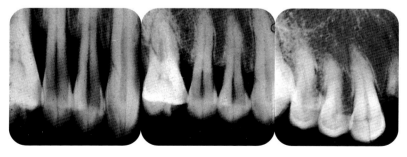

Fig 5-1 The effect of beam angulation in bisecting angle radiography on root length. The film in the centre was taken with the correct beam angulation, that on the left with too shallow an angle and that on the right with too steep an angle. The steep angle has also masked the periodontal bone loss.

The ideal periapical radiograph should display optimal image geometry and at least 3 mm of periapical bone to allow an adequate assessment of the apical status. Panoramic radiography is also used to assess periapical pathology although, as outlined in Chapter 4, the technique has severe limitations especially in the incisor, canine and premolar regions of the oral cavity.

Sensitivity values for periapical radiography in detecting apical change are high ranging from 65% to 84%. By comparison, panoramic radiography produces lower overall sensitivity levels falling to 29% for the mandibular incisor/canine region.

An effective way to identify the majority (90%) of apical lesions is by the use of referral criteria in combination with patients' clinical signs and symptoms and certain radiographic features (i.e. gross caries, previous endodontic therapy and heavily restored teeth) seen on bitewing radiographs. Panoramic or lateral oblique radiography may be useful in those patients with extensive inflammatory pathology.

Classification of Inflammatory Lesions

Inflammatory pathology will be discussed using the following headings.

periapical inflammatory disease
- chronic periapical periodontitis
- acute periapical periodontitis
- lesions associated with periapical periodontitis
pericoronitis
osteomyelitis
- acute osteomyelitis
- chronic osteomyelitis
     - chronic suppurative (or rarefying) osteomyelitis
     - sclerosing osteomyelitis
     - Garrè's osteomyelitis
osteoradionecrosis.

Periapical Inflammatory Disease

Pulpal necrosis represents the most common cause of changes to the periapical tissues. Periapical inflammation of pulp origin results in a variety of radiological signs that are summarised in Table 5-1.

Table 5-1. **The radiological signs associated with apical periodontitis.**

	Acute apical periodontitis	Chronic apical periodontitis
Loss of lamina dura	✓	
Widening of periapical periodontal ligament	✓	✓
Rarefying osteitis	✓	
Sclerosing osteitis		✓
Well-defined rounded radiolucency		✓

Chronic Periapical Periodontitis

Chronic periapical periodontitis represents a condition in which the inflammatory response is controlled by mechanisms within the host and is generally asymptomatic for the patient. The response of bone to low-grade and long-standing infection is specific and the radiological features are characteristic.

The following radiological signs are associated with the presence of low-grade chronic inflammation within the periapical tissues:
widening of the periodontal ligament space
widening of the periodontal ligament space and sclerosing (or condensing) osteitis
well-defined apical radiolucency.

Clinical features
The patient is usually asymptomatic or exhibits mild discomfort.

Radiological signs
The initial radiographic feature is a widening of the periodontal ligament space due to the accumulation of inflammatory exudate in the periapical tissue (Fig 5-2). The slow inflammatory process causes the remodelling of the lamina dura further from the tooth apex.

In the posterior maxilla, widening of the periodontal ligament space may

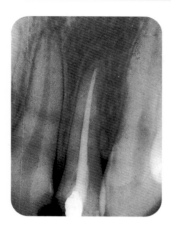

Fig 5-2 Widening of the periapical periodontal ligament on 22.

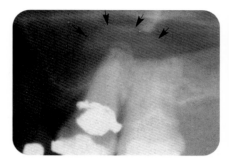

Fig 5-3 The first molar tooth has a widened periodontal ligament and an intact lamina dura. Above this the mucosa of the antral floor (arrowed) has thickened in response to the periapical inflammation, forming an "antral halo".

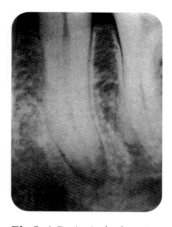

Fig 5-4 Periapical sclerosing (condensing) osteitis around a lower premolar.

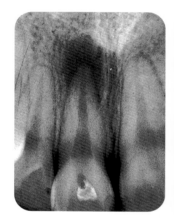

Fig 5-5 Periapical granuloma on 11. The radiolcency is well-defined and the lamina dura is absent from around the tooth apex.

elevate the antral floor. Periapical inflammatory toxins stimulate extra bone production and hypertrophy in the overlying antral mucosa (Fig 5-3). This appearance has been referred to as an "antral halo".

It is important to recognise that chronic periapical periodontitis can result in bone formation, in the form of a sclerosing (or condensing) osteitis (Fig 5-4). This appearance will often remain evident for many years subsequent to tooth extraction or successful endodontic therapy.

The development of a well-defined round apical radiolucency marks the development of a periapical granuloma (Fig 5-5) or a radicular cyst (see Chapter 9). Radiological differentiation between granuloma and cyst is related to the size of the lesion, but there is no clear cut-off point. A threshold of 10 mm is often given as a "rule of thumb" threshold. However, one-third of smaller radiolucencies will be cystic, while one-third of those with a diameter exceeding 15 mm will be granulomas. It is rare for a granuloma to exceed 20mm in diameter.

Acute Periapical Periodontitis

Acute periapical periodontitis may occur *de novo* or result as an acute exacerbation of an established chronic periapical periodontitis. Conversely, of course, an acute lesion can evolve into a chronic state. It is important to remember that no radiological features may be evident during the initial stages of the acute inflammatory episode, although the patient may be symptomatic.

The following radiological features are associated with the presence of acute inflammation within the periapical tissue and periapical bone:
• Loss of the lamina dura with/without widening of the periodontal ligament space.
• Rarefying osteitis (ill-defined diffuse radiolucency extending into surrounding bone).

Clinical features
The tooth is extremely sensitive to percussion. The patient complains of severe, constant pain and there may be associated soft tissue swelling.

Radiological signs
The earliest change is evidence of loss of the lamina dura at the apex and often a concurrent widening of the periodontal ligament space (Fig 5-6). With a rarefying osteitis, the radiological appearance is of an ill-defined radiolucency (Fig 5-7). A rarefying osteitis can present as an acute episode involving established chronic periapical lesions. Fig 5-8 shows a rarefying osteitis

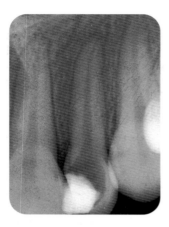

Fig 5-6 Loss of periapical lamina dura on 22.

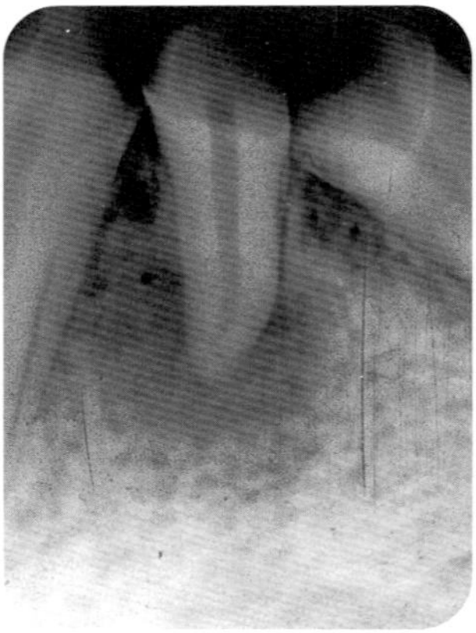

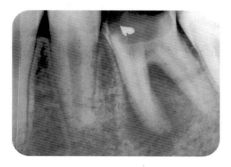

Fig 5-7 Periapical rarefying osteitis on the retained root. The margins of a radiolucency are diffuse (compare with the periapical granuloma in Fig 5-5).

Fig 5-8 Periapical rarefying osteitis with surrounding sclerosing osteitis on the carious 36.

where there is a surrounding sclerosing osteitis. In the case of acute inflammation arising in chronic apical granulomas and radicular cysts, there will be loss (either total or partial) of the well-defined peripheral margin and its replacement by ill-defined diffuse radiolucency.

Lesions Associated with Inflammation

External and internal resorption of teeth

Resorption of teeth is, of course, a normal physiological process that occurs in the deciduous dentition. The pathological process of resorption is, however, seen in association with inflammation. Pathological resorption can be divided into two types: external and internal.

- External resorption

External resorption commonly involves the root surface but can affect the crown of an unerupted tooth. The condition usually involves an individual tooth but occasional cases have been reported that involved the entire dentition. External resorption is a common sequel to pulpal infection. Other factors, however, have been recognised and are listed in Table 5-2.

Table 5-2. **Causes of external resorption and their radiological appearance**

Causes	Radiological appearance
Embedded teeth: most commonly canines and third molars	Completely embedded teeth affected. Resorption initiated on enamel surface at cemento-enamel junction and tooth tissue destroyed. Resorbing teeth show an ill-defined outline and a pronounced density reduction.
Fixed or removable orthodontic appliances	Resorption evident as blunted, shortened root apices of one or several teeth.
Adjacent mass: unerupted tooth (commonly upper canine, third molars) or adjacent benign mass (i.e. epithelium lined cyst, developmental lesion, osteosclerosis, ameloblastoma, giant cell tumour, cemento-osseous lesions).	There is a pronounced reduction in root length, but the resorbing root surface is well defined and may approximate exactly to the shape of the adjacent lesion.
Trauma, transplantation and reimplantation of avulsed teeth.	Resorption may be limited to a single site or in the case of transplantation and reimplantation teeth, the resorption is irregular and multiple sites of resorptive activity are usually evident.
Malignant lesions: malignant bone tumours, Langerhans' cell histiocytosis and metastatic deposits.	Ragged root resorption often associated with an encircling uniformly widened periodontal ligament space.

Clinical features

Non-specific pain or root fracture may be the presenting symptoms, but are restricted to advanced cases.

Radiological signs

External resorption can occur anywhere on the root surface. Apical resorption reduces root length and alters the root contour. Loss of the apical lamina dura invariably accompanies external resorption occurring as a result of apical infection (Fig 5-9).

Whilst resorption affecting the lateral and apical region of the tooth is readily identified, the presentation of resorption affecting the buccal or lingual root surface is more challenging. In external resorption, the linear radiopaque lines demarcating the root canal are retained (Fig 5-10), at least until the resorption is extensive. This is due to the fact that the dentine adjacent to the pulp is very resistant to resorption and, therefore, this radiological sign tends to persist. Parallax is useful in determining the exact position of the area of resorption.

- Internal resorption

Internal resorption occurs within the pulp chamber or canal and results in resorption of the adjacent dentine and enlargement of the pulp. The aetiol-

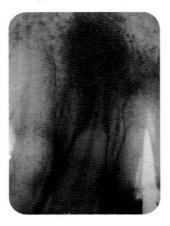

Fig 5-9 Apical external resorption in association with a periapical inflammatory lesion.

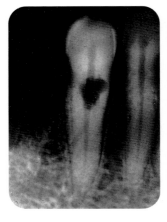

Fig 5-10 External resorption "en face" on 43. The outline of the root canal is still visible.

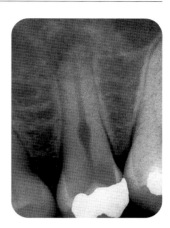

Fig 5-11 Internal resorption. A short length of canal is widened, with no sign of the outline of the original canal. There is also a periapical granuloma.

ogy is unknown, although pulpal inflammation and trauma have been implicated.

Clinical features
In most cases, the condition is asymptomatic. In advanced cases, the first evidence of the lesion may be a "pink spot" on the crown or when the lesion is localised to the root, a pathological fracture or pulpitis.

Radiological signs
The radiological picture is localised enlargement of the pulp chamber or root canal (Fig 5-11). The margin of the lesion is well defined but with a variable shape. There is loss of the original outline of the pulp canal that differentiates this lesion from external resorption.

Hypercementosis

Hypercementosis is an increase in the thickness of the cementum and can occur in relation to chronic periapical inflammation. However, it is also seen with periodontal disease (see Chapter 4) and in association with Paget's disease (Chapter 10).

Radiological signs
There is pronounced thickening of cementum, most commonly in and around the apical region, giving the root a bulbous appearance (Fig 5-12).

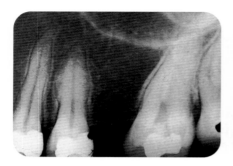 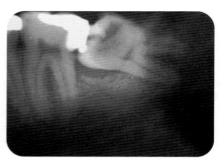

Fig 5-12 Hypercementosis affecting 25.

Fig 5-13 This impacted carious 38 had undergone repeated episodes of pericoronal infection. Note the subtle increase in bone density deep to the pericoronal space.

Pericoronitis

This is inflammation surrounding the crown of an unerupted tooth, most commonly a lower third molar in a young adult.

Clinical features
Pain and swelling related to the operculum over the crown of the tooth. There may be traumatic occlusion from an overerupted upper molar.

Radiological signs
The changes depend on the longevity of the condition. Where pericoronitis has been recurrent, the commonest signs are of an enlarged pericoronal space with a peripheral sclerosing (condensing) osteitis (Figs 5-13 and 8-16).

Osteomyelitis

Osteomyelitis is an inflammatory disease of the bone and bone marrow. It develops subsequent to dental or other types of infection and is more commonly found in the mandible. Conditions that predispose to the development of osteomyelitis are:
- diabetes (poorly controlled)
- blood dyscrasias - anaemia, neutropaenia, sickle cell anaemia
- bone abnormalities- Paget's disease of bone, osteopetrosis, gigantiform cementoma
- altered host resistance.

Clinically, the disease presents in an acute or a chronic form. Acute osteomyelitis may produce little or no radiographic evidence of disease, whereas in chronic osteomyelitis radiological features are consistently seen.

Acute osteomyelitis
Clinical features
The condition presents rapidly with pain and swelling of adjacent soft tissue and accompanying lymphadenopathy. Involved teeth may be tender to percussion and the patient may report altered sensation (paraesthesia).

Radiological signs
In the initial stages, radiographic examination will reveal either no change or be limited to a rarefying osteitis. If the lesion involves the cortices of the jaw and/or the mandibular canal, the margins of these structures will appear indistinct. Similarly, involved teeth will lose their lamina dura.

Chronic osteomyelitis
Chronic osteomyelitis presents radiographically in several ways, each representing a variation in the response of bone to infection. Three distinct subtypes can be identified:
- Chronic suppurative (or rarefying) osteomyelitis
- Sclerosing osteomyelitis
- Garrè's osteomyelitis

Chronic suppurative (or rarefying) osteomyelitis
The disease can occur *de novo* or represent a progression from the acute stage into a chronic form.

Clinical features
The patient will give a history of symptoms continuing over several weeks and report episodes of pain and swelling and lymphadenopathy in the jaws. There is usually evidence of sinus formation and the patient may report altered sensation.

Radiological signs
The periphery of the lesion may be irregular and ill-defined or, in more established cases, a peripheral sclerosis may be seen separating normal from infected bone. Adjacent teeth, if involved in the inflammatory process, will show loss of the lamina dura. The involved bone shows ill-defined patchy radiolucency separated by loci of apparently "normal" bone. As the disease

progresses, these radiolucent areas will coalesce and enlarge (Fig 5-14), often involving the cortex of the bone. The dense radiopacities are islands of non-vital necrotic bone or *sequestra* (Fig 5-15). The disease can induce new bone formation, a process referred to as *proliferative periostitis* or *involucrum* formation. This is seen as one or more radiopaque lines parallel to the cortex and to each other (Fig 5-16).

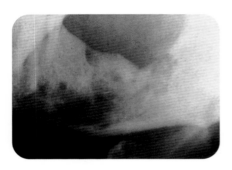

Fig 5-14 Chronic osteomyelitis of the mandible, extending to involve the lower border. The jaw is "moth eaten" in appearance.

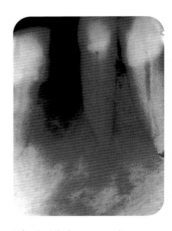

Fig 5-15 Sequestra in osteomyelitis affecting the anterior mandible following extraction of 31 two weeks previously. Note that the sequestra lie deeply, surrounded by a rarefying osteitis. Compare this with the appearance of a "socket sequestrum" (Fig 10-5).

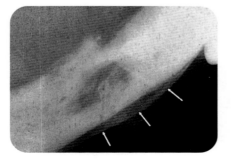

Fig 5-16 Periosteal new bone. This is an occlusal radiograph of the 46 region. The body of the mandible is occupied by an area of bone destruction due to osteomyelitis, with cortical perforation lingually. On the buccal aspect the layer of new bone is arrowed.

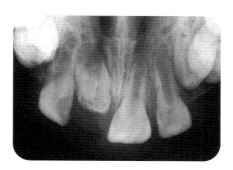

Fig 6-2 Turner's hypoplasia affecting an unerupted 11. The crown is pitted. There was a history of previous chronic abscess on the deciduous precursor.

Clinical features

Permanent incisors or premolars are affected. The degree of hypoplasia depends upon the stage of tooth development and the severity and extent of the infection or trauma. Similar appearances can be seen affecting the developing teeth of children who have undergone radiotherapy to the head and neck region.

Radiological signs

If the deformity is minimal, the tooth will show a localised area of hypoplasia. A prolonged disturbance will lead to pronounced changes in tooth morphology that include gross deformity, irregularity and a reduction in crown size (Fig 6-2).

Amelogenesis Imperfecta

This is an inherited condition affecting enamel formation in both dentitions. From a purely radiological standpoint, amelogenesis imperfecta can be classified into two types: *hypoplastic* and *hypocalcified*.

Hypoplastic amelogenesis imperfecta

This occurs during the early stage of enamel formation and results in an abnormal enamel matrix that subsequently undergoes normal mineralisation.

Clinical features

The enamel matrix is either extremely thin or absent, with a variable appearance described as pitted, smooth, rough or glossy. The crowns of the teeth are "square-shaped", resembling a tooth prepared for a full coronal restoration.

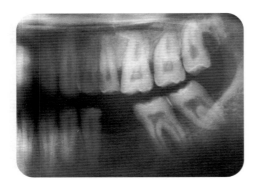

Fig 6-3 Hypoplastic amelogenesis imperfecta. Note the thin enamel but normal underlying tooth structure.

Radiological signs
The enamel is extremely thin but with a normal radiopacity compared to the underlying dentine (Fig 6-3).

Hypocalcified amelogenesis imperfecta
This represents disturbances occurring later in enamel formation affecting either the maturation or mineralisation of the matrix. The enamel has a normal thickness but defective mineralisation.

Clinical features
The colour of the affected crown ranges from clear through to brown. The enamel fractures away easily resulting in rapid attrition and a reduction in tooth height.

Radiological signs
There is a lack of radiographic contrast between dentine and enamel.

Anomalies of Dentine: Generalised

Dentinogenesis imperfecta
Dentinogenesis imperfecta, an inherited condition, affects both dentitions and is classified into two main types. In Type I, the condition coexists with osteogenesis imperfecta. In Type II there are no associated skeletal abnormalities.

Clinical features
The appearance of the teeth is characteristic, having an opalescent hue and small size. The enamel readily fractures from the tooth resulting in rapid attrition.

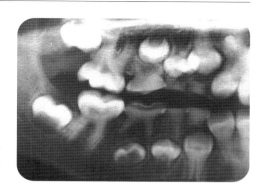

Fig 6-4 Dentinogenesis imperfecta. The bulbous crowns and spindly roots are typical features.

Radiological signs
The crowns of the teeth have a pronounced cervical constriction giving a "bulbous" appearance (Fig 6-4). There is obliteration of the pulp. The roots are short and slender and root fractures have been reported. Periapical radiolucencies are seen.

Dentinal dysplasia
Dentinal dysplasia is an inherited condition affecting both dentitions. It is divided into two types: Type I (radicular dentinal dysplasia) and Type II (coronal dentinal dysplasia). It occurs less frequently than dentinogenesis imperfecta.

Clinical features
Type I is the more frequent type. Teeth erupt normally with no obvious abnormality but rapidly develop mobility resulting from limited root support. In type II, the deciduous teeth are similar to those in dentinogenesis imperfecta, whereas the permanent teeth appear normal.

Radiological signs
In Type I, all the teeth, except the canines, have extremely short roots. The roots are conical or blunted. There is pulpal obliteration and the inferior aspects of the crown exhibit linear crescent-shaped radiolucent lines. Periapical radiolucencies are commonly seen associated with non-carious teeth in Type I dentinal dysplasia. In Type II dentinal dysplasia, obliteration of the pulp occurs post eruption in the deciduous dentition. In the permanent dentition, there is alteration in the configuration of the pulp resulting in enlarged pulp chambers extending well down into the root (Fig 6-5). The pulp contains multiple calcifications.

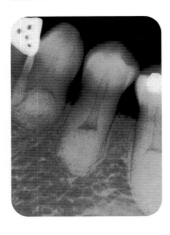

Fig 6-5 Type II dentinal dysplasia. All of this patient's teeth were similarly affected.

Anomalies of Enamel and Dentine

Regional odontodysplasia
Regional odontodysplasia is a rare defect characterised by hypoplastic and hypomineralised enamel and dentine. The pathogenesis is unknown.

Clinical features
The condition is found in both dentitions and usually localised to a few adjacent teeth. The maxilla and the anterior regions of the jaws appear to be more commonly affected. The involved teeth may show delayed eruption or a failure to erupt. If eruption occurs, the degree of abnormality is obvious.

Radiological signs
There is a marked reduction in the radiopacity of the dental tissue giving the teeth a "ghost-like" appearance. It is impossible to differentiate enamel from dentine. The pulp chamber and canal(s) appear large and the root length shortened (Fig 6-6).

Altered Crown Morphology

Dens invaginatus
This anomaly is the result of an infolding of the enamel organ prior to calcification and represents, in its coronal form, an accentuation of the cingulum pit. The anomaly is believed to be genetically determined and has a prevalence of 5%. The maxillary lateral incisors are commonly affected. The condition rarely occurs in the deciduous dentition.

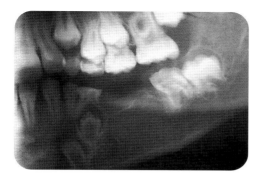

Fig 6-6 Regional odontodysplasia showing the "ghost teeth" appearance of developing teeth in the lower-left quadrant.

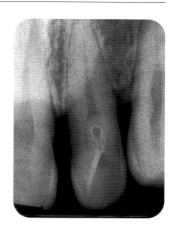

Fig 6-7 Dens invaginatus affecting 22. Note that the pit is lined with a thin enamel layer. The pulp bifurcates around the pit.

Clinical features
The condition is asymptomatic. The clinical appearance of the cingulum may be normal or display a deepened cingulum pit.

Radiological signs
The invagination appears as a linear radiopacity at the level of the cingulum. It varies in the degree that it involves the coronal tooth tissue (Fig 6-7). The tooth may display an open apex and periapical radiolucency as a sequel to loss of pulp vitality.

Anomalies of the Pulp/Root Canals

Reduction of size
This is a normal ageing process but may be associated with dental caries, large restorations, erosion, attrition or abrasion.

Pulp Stones/Pulp Sclerosis

See Chapter 2 pages 19—20.

Altered Root Morphology

Taurodontism
Taurodontism is an inherited abnormality occurring either as an isolated trait or rarely in association with certain syndromes. It affects molar and premolar teeth.

Radiological signs
The pulp chamber extends well below the cementoenamel junction and has a rectangular form due to the absence of a normal cervical constriction. Furcation of the root occurs at a shortened distance above the root apex (Fig 6-8).

Supernumerary Roots

This condition is not rare and may involve any tooth. Teeth commonly affected include the mandibular canine, maxillary second premolar and mandibular first molar.

Radiological signs
Supernumerary roots are diagnosed by radiography (Fig 6-9). An accurate radiological diagnosis often requires the use of parallax techniques.

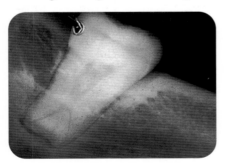

Fig 6-8 Taurodont 47. The pulp chamber is greatly elongated and the root canals correspondingly short.

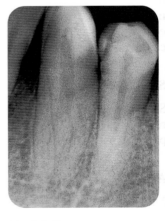

Fig 6-9 Supernumerary root on 33.

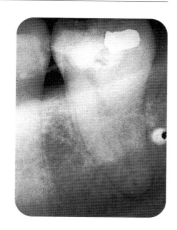

Fig 6-10 Apical dilaceration of 38, with a "bull's eye" appearance at the apex.

Dilacerated Root

Dilaceration represents a sharp bend in the root surface. Maxillary incisors, maxillary premolars and mandibular third molars are commonly affected. A severe defect may result in non-eruption of the involved tooth.

Radiological signs

Mesial and distal dilacerations are readily apparent radiographically. Bucco-palatal/lingual displacement of the root presents as a "bull's-eye" comprising the superimposition of the root apex surrounded peripherally by the periodontal ligament space and the lamina dura with the radiolucency of the root canal positioned centrally (Fig 6-10).

Shortened Roots

Shortened roots occurring with normal crown morphology are usually the result of disturbed root formation (e.g. due to radiotherapy or surgery) or particular syndromes (dentinal dysplasia or dentinogenesis imperfecta).

Alteration in Tooth Size

Macrodontia

Tooth size is genetically determined with males having larger teeth than females. True macrodontia may occur in pituitary gigantism and hemihypertrophy of the face. Relative macrodontia is more common, occurring when normal teeth are seen in a small jaw. Gemination and fusion present clinically as large teeth.

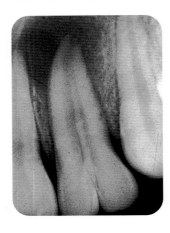

Fig 6-11 Gemination of 22. There is also a large periapical granuloma.

Gemination
Gemination is an attempt by the developing tooth to divide producing a widened crown with an incisal notch. It occurs more commonly in the anterior maxilla and in the deciduous dentition. There is a normal compliment of teeth.

Radiological signs
The tooth has a notched incisal margin with a confluent or partially joined pulp canal system (Fig 6-11).

Fusion
Fusion is the union between dentine and enamel of two or more separate developing teeth. Anterior teeth are more often affected. Fusion is more common in the deciduous dentition. The number of teeth present is reduced by one, unless fusion involves a supernumerary tooth.

Radiological signs
The tooth has a notched incisal margin and there is evidence of conjoined dentine between the involved teeth (Fig 6-12). The fused tooth may present with two distinct pulp chambers/pulp canal systems or a joined system.

Microdontia
Microdontia is a term used to describe teeth that are smaller than normal. True microdontia is extremely rare and may be seen in pituitary dwarfism, Down's syndrome and as a feature of dentinogenesis imperfecta. In relative microdontia, the teeth are normal but in a larger than normal jaw. Microdon-

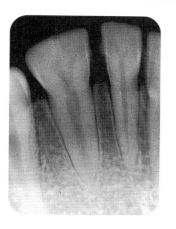

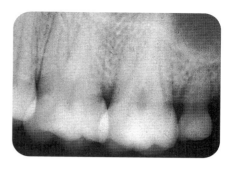

Fig 6-13 Microdontia. This third molar is considerably smaller than normal. 61

Fig 6-12 Fusion of 41 and 42.

tia can be limited to individual teeth, as evidenced by "peg-shaped" lateral incisors, diminutive third molars (Fig 6-13) and supernumerary teeth (see below).

Altered Tooth Morphology

Dens in dente and the dilated odontomes
The dens in dente and the dilated odontome are a result of infolding of the enamel organ and represent more severe forms of dens invaginatus (see above). These anomalies are found more commonly in the anterior regions.

Radiological signs
Dens in dente represents a tooth-shaped, enamel-covered mass within the crown and/or root of the tooth but which may traverse the length of the tooth (Fig 6-14). Dilated odontome represents the most extreme form of this anomaly and exhibits a grossly altered morphology that is internally outlined by a dense linear radiopacity (Fig 6-15). In both cases, the apical region may or may not display an open apex and there may be associated adjacent apical rarefaction.

Anomalies Affecting the Number of Teeth

Missing teeth
A congenital absence of teeth may be total *(anodontia)* or partial *(hypodontia)*.

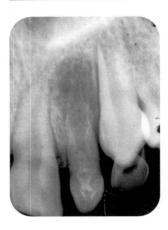

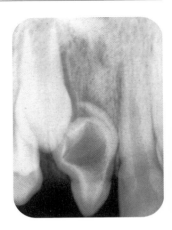

Fig 6-14 Dens-in-dente. This tooth was ostensibly a "peg lateral". However, radiography revealed a deep enamel lined pit extending into the pulp. The apex is incomplete and there is a periapical granuloma.

Fig 6-15 Dilated odontome. This anomaly of 12 can be seen as an extreme version of dens-in-dente. The large radiolucency centrally, lined with enamel, is the pit. The pulp is the crescent-shaped radiolucency lying deep to this.

Anodontia is extremely rare. Hypodontia is more common but usually limited to the permanent dentition. Radiotherapy to the jaws can destroy the developing tooth bud with consequent hypodontia.

Clinical features

The following are most commonly affected: third molars, maxillary lateral incisors, mandibular second premolars and mandibular central incisors. These teeth may be missing symmetrically or unilaterally. In the deciduous dentition, the maxillary lateral and mandibular central and lateral incisors are most frequently absent. Prolonged retention of deciduous teeth or the presence of an ankylosed, submerging second deciduous molar should alert the clinician to the possibility of hypodontia.

Radiological signs

Hypodontia (Fig 6-16) is definitively diagnosed radiologically by the absence of a tooth at a time after the normal date of tooth crypt formation has passed (see Chapter 2).

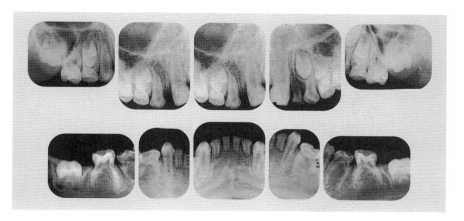

Fig 6-16 Hypodontia. In the mandible the only permanent teeth in development are 36 and 46. In the maxilla there are a few more permanent teeth: 16, 14, 11, 21, 23, 24 and 26.

Additional Teeth (Hyperdontia)

Hyperdontia is considered an inherited trait. It is rarely found in the deciduous dentition. It may occur alone or in association with developmental abnormalities (cleft palate) and syndromes (cleidocranial dysplasia, Gardner's and Ehlers–Danlos). Teeth with morphological features identical to the normal standing tooth are known as *supplemental* teeth and those with an abnormal and diminutive form are referred to as *supernumerary* teeth. The latter are given a further sub-classification according to their position in the jaws:

- *mesiodens*: positioned between the maxillary central incisors.
- *distodens*: positioned distal to the third molars.
- *paramolar*: positioned buccal or palatal to the maxillary molars.

Clinical features

The detection of erupted additional teeth is uncomplicated. The presence of additional teeth may be indirectly inferred as a result of a missing or a misaligned tooth in the dental arch. In these cases, radiography forms an essential component of diagnosis and treatment planning.

Radiological signs

Supplemental teeth are commonly found in the mandibular second premolar region (Fig 6-17), the maxillary lateral incisor region and the mandibular

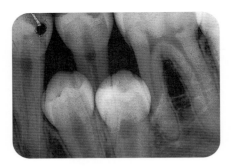

Fig 6-17 Supplemental lower-left premolars.

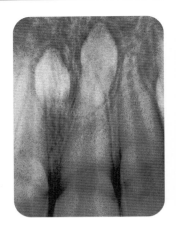

Fig 6-18 Supernumerary teeth. There are two "mesiodens" supernumeraries, both inverted.

central incisor region. *Supernumerary* teeth are generally conical in shape and are found in specific areas in the jaws outlined above (Fig 6-18).

All types of additional teeth appear as a dense radiopacity. They can undergo cystic change and may cause resorption of adjacent teeth. The *mesiodens* may be conical or tuberculate in form, with the former usually displacing incisors whilst the latter prevents their eruption.

Further Reading

Langland OE, Langlais RP. Principles of Dental Imaging. 2nd ed. Philadelphia: Lippincott Williams and Wilkins, 1997: 375-394.

Taybi H. Handbook of Syndromes and Metabolic Disorders: Radiologic and Clinical Manifestations. Mosby, St Louis; 1998.

Whaites E. Developmental abnormalities. In: Whaites E. Essentials of Dental Radiography and Radiology. 3rd ed. Edinburgh: Churchill Livingstone, 2002: 261-270.

White SC and Pharoah MJ. Dental Anomalies. In: White SC, Pharoah MJ (Eds.) Oral Radiology. Principles and Interpretation. 4th ed. St Louis: Mosby, 2000: 303-337.

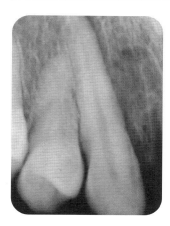

Fig 7-2 Periapical radiograph showing a slightly luxated 13. It has been displaced buccally, appears elongated, and there is a widened periodontal ligament space mesially.

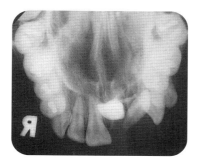

Fig 7-3 Occlusal view showing luxation of upper left incisor teeth. Because 21 is retroclined, the x-ray beam passes down its long axis, so it appears in plan view and very dense. Note also that the 22 has also been markedly displaced.

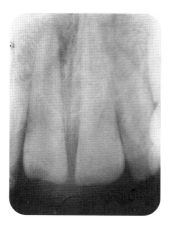

Fig 7-4 Periapical radiograph of severely intruded teeth. Note how the incisal edges of the central incisors are more apically positioned than those of the adjacent upper left lateral incisors. The central incisor crowns are covered by soft tissue swelling and blood clot and thus are not so clearly visible.

Fractures of the crown

Coronal fracture (Fig 7-6) is largely a matter of clinical examination. Radiography serves a useful purpose in demonstrating the location of the pulp relative to the fracture. It is not, however, always possible to determine from the radiograph whether the pulp is involved; this is a clinical diagnosis.

It is important to be able to account for any missing crown fragments. In some cases, a portion of the fractured crown becomes embedded within the soft tis-

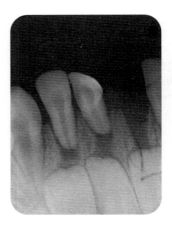

Fig 7-5 Extrusion of both right primary incisors and avulsion of the lower-left central incisor. The partly empty radiolucent sockets are clearly seen, just above the permanent incisors.

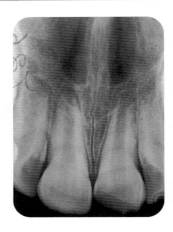

Fig 7-6 Fracture of the crown of the mandibular left incisor, involving the enamel and dentine but not the pulp.

sues of the lips. When this is suspected (because of soft tissue laceration and swelling of the lip), radiographic views of the lips should be taken to confirm the presence of the foreign body. A useful initial view is that of a soft-tissue lateral of the lips taken using an occlusal film, placed parallel to the sagittal plane against the side of the face but in line with the lips. The exposure time should be reduced by approximately 25% compared to that given for a normal upper incisor radiograph, to show the soft tissue profile. This view (Fig 7-7) will confirm the presence and depth of the foreign body and a decision can be made whether further views are required. A complementary radiograph is produced by exposing a periapical film in the labial sulcus, again using a soft tissue (reduced) exposure (Fig 7-8).

Fractures of the root
Accidental fractures of the root occur less commonly than do those of the crown, accounting for up to 7% of injuries affecting the permanent dentition and up to 4% of the primary dentition. Root fractures mainly affect the upper incisors and are unlikely to occur to teeth whose roots have not fully formed.
A radiographic examination is needed to confirm the presence and site of a root fracture. The radiographic appearance of a fractured root is that of a radiolucent line (or lines) running across the root. Widening of the fracture

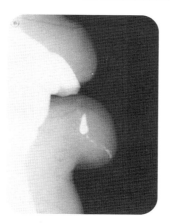

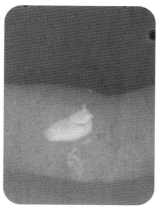

Fig 7-7 Soft tissue view showing a fragment of an upper central incisor crown, side on, embedded in the lower lip. The injury is a through and through one (i.e. the crown has penetrated completely through the lip), as indicated by the tract left by fragments of the splintered crown.

Fig 7-8 Soft tissue of the lower lip taken at right angles to that in Fig 7-7, showing the fractured crown face on.

line indicates separation of the fractured fragments. How well the fracture is seen on the radiograph depends on the direction of the fracture to the incident x-ray beam and the degree of separation of the root fragments.

A fracture will be seen as a single radiolucent line when the x-ray beam passes along the fracture (Figs 7-9a and 7-9b), particularly if there is separation of the fractured portions. If, however, the fracture plane is oblique to the x-ray beam, the root fracture may appear as a double fracture line (Figs 7-10a and 7-10b). The clinical case in both figures is the same one; the different radiological appearance reflects the steeper x-ray beam angulation in Fig 7-9.

The cases shown in Figs 7-11, 7-12 and 7-13 illustrate the variable appearances of root fractures.

Root fracture is a complication of post crown restorations. In this case, the fracture tends to run in a vertical direction. Detection of the fracture can be difficult where a radiopaque metal post obscures it. Loss of the lamina dura and a laterally positioned radiolucency in a patient with a post crown is a useful radiological sign when looking for a suspected root fracture, as it indicates the presence of inflammation at the site of the fracture (Fig 7-14).

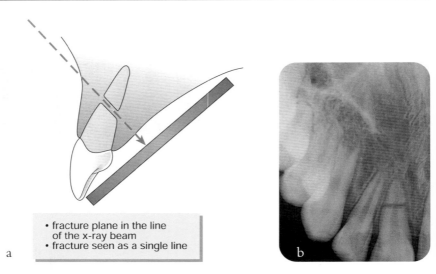

- fracture plane in the line
  of the x-ray beam
- fracture seen as a single line

a

b

Fig 7-9 Root fracture of 11. Line diagram (a) and radiograph (b), explaining why a root fracture may appear as a single line.

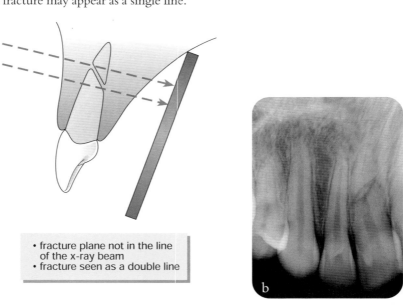

- fracture plane not in the line
  of the x-ray beam
- fracture seen as a double line

a

b

Fig 7-10 Root fracture of 11. Line diagram (a) and radiograph (b), explaining why a root fracture may appear as a double line. The radiograph is, in fact, of the same patient as in Fig 7-9.

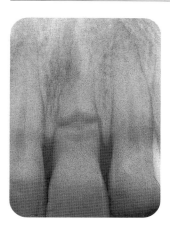

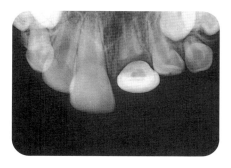

Fig 7-12 Coronal third root fracture of 21 with palatal displacement of the coronal fragment.

Fig 7-11 Comminuted root fracture of 21, in which a slither of root can be seen in the middle of the fracture.

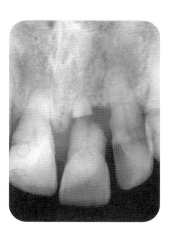

Fig 7-13 Root fracture in 21 in a patient with periodontal bone loss. The fracture has occurred at the alveolar bone level, which has acted as a fulcrum.

Sequelae of Tooth Trauma

Patients who have traumatised their teeth should be followed up clinically and radiographically to assess the success of treatment. The sequelae include:
* Failure of completion of root development (Figs 7-15 and 7-16).
* Periapical inflammation (Fig 7-16).
* Resorption (Figs 7-15 and 7-17).
* Ankylosis (Fig 7-17).

Teeth that have been reimplanted or surgically transplanted may undergo ankylosis or resorption. Where ankylosis occurs there is loss of the periodontal ligament space, so that the root abuts against the bone. The radi-

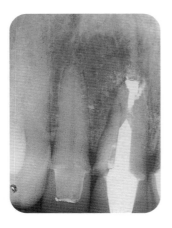

Fig 7-14 Vertical root fracture of 11. The fracture is noticeable because there is displacement of the fractured distal portion. The fracture runs down the distal aspect of the post where there is separation between it and root, after which the fracture becomes more oblique. At the point where the fracture ends short of below the apex, there is loss of lamina dura and a small area of radiolucency.

ographic features of resorption have been described in Chapter 5. Teeth that have been surgically transplanted are prone to resorption and ankylosis.

Fractures Involving Bone

Dentoalveolar fractures

A dentoalveolar fracture is a localised fracture involving a segment of the alveolus. There is usually intraoral bleeding of the gingivae or oral mucosa. If the fractured fragment is displaced there will be an altered occlusion.

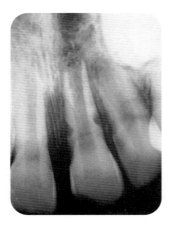

Fig 7-15 Mesial and distal resorption cavities on a reimplanted 21. The tooth was avulsed and reimplanted whilst it still had an open apex and, as a result of this injury, root development ceased. Where there has been instrumentation on the root surface, mesial and distal resorption cavities have formed.

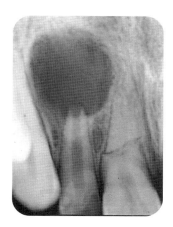

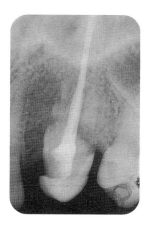

Fig 7-16 Radiograph of a 19-year-old showing a healed root fracture of 11 and arrested root development of 12. The trauma had occurred at the age of 10 years. A radicular cyst has developed on 12.

Fig 7-17 Root resorption and ankylosis affecting a maxillary canine surgically transplanted over 10 years previously. There is extensive external root resorption. Ankylosis is shown by the partial loss of the periodontal ligament space.

Movement of one tooth usually results in movement of the other tooth or teeth on that fragment.

As with fractures of the teeth, dentoalveolar fractures are seen as radiolucent lines, and their clarity will depend upon the direction of the x-ray beam to the plane of the fracture and upon whether the fracture is displaced. The fracture may be less obvious if the x-ray beam passes across or is oblique to the fracture line, particularly if there is minimal displacement of the fracture. Fig 7-18 shows a minimally displaced dento-alveolar fracture of the mandible, while Fig 7-19 shows a more extensive fracture in the maxilla.

Fracture of the maxillary tuberosity

This is an uncommon event, but is most likely to occur when extracting a single standing upper second or third molar tooth. Following extraction of upper molar teeth, the alveolus often becomes pneumatised by the maxillary antrum. This leaves relatively weak bony walls that are prone to fracture during the extraction of any remaining molar tooth. When the tuberosity

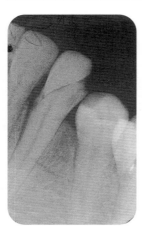

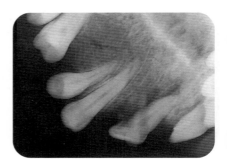

Fig 7-18 Dentoalveolar fracture lower-left canine / premolar region. The crown of 33 is also fractured. Running between this tooth and the first premolar is a thin radiolucent line which represents the bony fracture.

Fig 7-19 Dentoalveolar fracture of maxilla running from the upper right central incisor to the upper right first molar. The fracture line is not straight but starts close to the alveolar crest just distal to the upper incisor and runs upwards and backwards just above the apices of the premolar and then downwards to the periodontal ligament space of the upper first molar. Note that there is also lateral luxation of 11.

fractures, there is a sudden "give" and the tooth with its investing buccal, palatal and distal bone will move as one. The value of radiography is not so much to diagnose the fracture, but to demonstrate the position of the antral floor to the fracture and the tooth (Fig 7-20).

Fracture of the genial tubercles
This is an uncommon fracture and is only seen where there has been marked alveolar bone resorption. The condition may be asymptomatic or the patient may have discomfort just lingual to the mandibular midline. Palpation reveals a hard, bony fragment in the region of the submandibular duct orifices. The area may be tender, but often the patient is symptom free. The radiological picture is demonstrated by Fig 7-21.

Fracture of the mandible
A clinical examination may show facial swelling, an altered occlusion or a step deformity, some degree of trismus and there may be sensory deficit

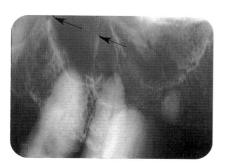

Fig 7-20 Radiograph of a fractured maxillary tuberosity. The main finding is discontinuity of the cortical lines of the maxillary sinus wall and septa (arrowed), as the fragment has been inferiorly displaced. 18 and 17 are included on the fragment.

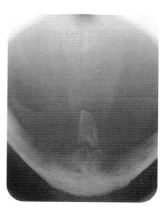

Fig 7-21 Fracture of the genial tubercles. The genial tubercles lie medial to their normal position.

affecting the mental region. There is nearly always tenderness on digital pressure at the fracture site(s) and this is a useful pointer when examining the radiograph for the location of a fracture. Thus, the mandible should be palpated from condyle to condyle, the occlusion should be examined for premature contacts, the teeth examined for possible fractures and the soft tissue inspected for injury.

The key radiological signs are:
- radiolucent line(s)
- radiopaque band(s)
- step deformity
- "displaced" anatomy
- soft tissue swelling.

It is important to remember that mandibular fractures are often bilateral. Thus, when one fracture is discovered on the radiograph, a search should be made for others, particularly on the contralateral side.

A simple crack fracture appears as a radiolucent line. The appearance of this type of fracture depends on the direction of the x-ray beam to the direction of the fracture. If the beam passes along the fracture plane it appears a single fracture line (Fig 7-22). However, if the fracture runs oblique to the beam, two fracture lines are seen. This is because most of the radiodensity of bone comes from the dense cortical plates, rather than the cancellous bone. So although there is just one fracture, each fractured cortical plate (buccal and lingual) is visible on the radiograph (Fig 7-23). The two fracture lines will, however, join somewhere along their length as they become superimposed upon one another, usually at the alveolar crest and lower border of the mandible. Radiopaque "bands" reflect a situation where two fractured bone ends are overlapped. The x-ray beam passes through two bone thicknesses, producing a radiopacity. A displaced fracture (Fig 7-24) is easy to identify because of the obvious gap between the bone ends.

A common site for a fracture is at, or on either side of, the midline. DPRs do not always display this region clearly (Fig 7-25). Suspected fractures at this site are better demonstrated on intraoral views, such as a lower anterior occlusal.

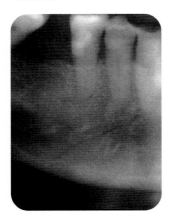

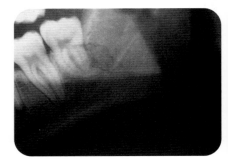

Fig 7-22 Fracture of the mandible running from 43 to the lower border. There is just a fine radiolucent line representing the undisplaced fracture.

Fig 7-23 Undisplaced mandibular fracture at the left angle, showing two radiolucent lines representing the break in the buccal and lingual cortices.

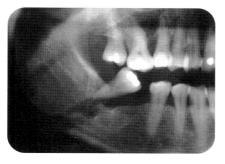

Fig 7-24 Mandibular fracture running through the molar tooth socket. There is marked upward displacement of the posterior fragment.

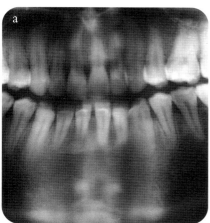
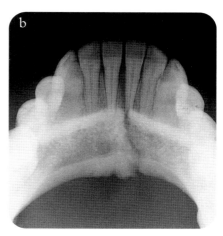

Fig 7-25 This midline fracture is not seen on the panoramic film (a) but is obvious on the lower anterior occlusal view (b).

Further Reading

Andreasen JO, Andreasen FM. Textbook and Color Atlas of Traumatic Injuries to the Teeth. 3rd ed. St Louis: Mosby, 1994.

Curzon MEJ. Handbook of Dental Trauma: A Practical Guide to the Treatment of Trauma to the Teeth. Bristol: Wright, 1999.

Roberts GJ, Longhurst P. Oral and Dental Trauma in Children and Adolescence. Oxford: Oxford University Press, 1996.

White SC, Pharoah MJ. Trauma to teeth and facial structures. In: White SC, Pharoah MJ (Eds.) Oral Radiology. Principles and Interpretation. 4th ed. St Louis: Mosby, 2000: 566-587.

Chapter 8

Assessment of Roots and Unerupted Teeth

Aim

The aim of this chapter is to outline the important radiographic features in the assessment of retained roots and unerupted teeth and the appropriate choice of radiographs. Emphasis is placed on those teeth that most commonly fail fully to erupt, mandibular third molars and maxillary canines, and on the assessment of retained roots.

Introduction

It is common for one or more of the permanent teeth to fail fully to erupt. This may be due to insufficient space to accommodate the erupting tooth or because eruption is impeded, for example, by the presence of a supernumerary tooth or a pathological lesion such as a cyst or tumour. More rarely, failure of eruption is seen in systemic conditions, such as cleidocranial dysplasia and Gardner's Syndrome (see Chapters 6 and 10). Although any tooth may fail to erupt, the commonest ones to do so are mandibular third molars and maxillary canines.

Choice of Radiographs

In the case of a suspected unerupted tooth or retained root, it is important first to undertake a clinical history and examination. The location and number of unerupted teeth determine the need for, and type of, radiographic examination. Where several teeth or roots are thought to be unerupted, especially in more than one quadrant, a DPR is more suitable than several periapical views. Selected periapical radiographs can then be taken if the roots or teeth are not clearly shown. In those cases where an unerupted tooth is deeply buried, a periapical radiograph may not show the full extent of the tooth. In such circumstances, a larger film such as an occlusal, oblique lateral or sectional DPR may be more appropriate.

Mandibular Third Molars

Impacted third molars should only be removed provided there is a valid clin-

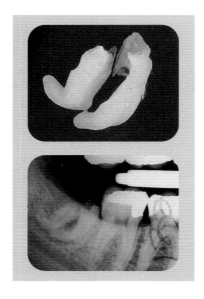

Fig 8-1 No radiograph had been taken prior to the attempted extraction of this lower third molar. Consequently, the operator was unaware of the hooked roots, which resulted in root fracture during extraction.

ical reason for doing so. In the UK, National Guidelines have been produced to assist the clinician with the decision whether third molar removal is required. Most guidelines suggest that wisdom teeth should not be removed unless there is a valid clinical reason for doing so, such as repeated episodes of pericoronitis or unrestorable dental decay of the third molar.

Third molars should always be radiographed prior to removal, even when fully erupted, because of the relative frequency of variable root morphology (Fig 8-1). In addition, it is important to be aware of the proximity of the roots of lower third molars to the mandibular canal. Such a situation may be present even with a fully erupted molar.

All unerupted or partly erupted teeth should be assessed in a logical and thorough manner, noting the depth, angulation, root morphology and proximity to other structures such as the mandibular canal and, in the case of an upper third molar, to the floor of the maxillary antrum.

Routine radiographic examination of unerupted third molars is not recommended.

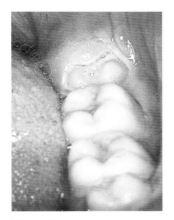

Fig 8-2 A partly erupted lower-left third molar.

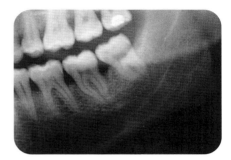

Fig 8-3 Radiograph of the patient shown in Fig 8-2.

Radiographic Assessment of Mandibular Third Molars

Type and angulation of the impaction

The tooth can be classified as a *soft tissue*, a *tooth*, a *bone* impaction, or a combination thereof. Figs. 8-2 and 8-3 show a soft tissue impaction. The clinical photograph (Fig 8-2) shows the partly erupted lower left third molar to lie vertically and the distal part of the crown to be covered by an operculum. The radiograph (Fig 8-3) confirms the vertical orientation and shows that the crown tooth is not impacted against tooth mesially nor bone, distally. Its only impaction is that of the soft tissue operculum.

The impaction can also be described by the angulation the tooth adopts in relation to the lower second molar. These are:
• horizontal
• mesioangular
• vertical
• distoangular
• transverse (rarely).

An example of a transversely impacted third molar is shown in Fig 8-4. Its presence on the bitewing radiograph was an unexpected finding. Fig 8-5 shows a distoangular impaction.

The crown

In most cases the presence of caries dictates that the third molar should be

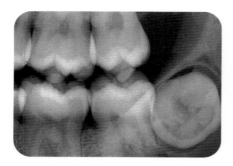 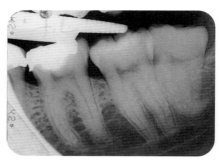

Fig 8-4 Transversely impacted lower third molar. In this situation, a lower true occlusal radiograph would help determine whether the crown is buccally or lingually displaced.

Fig 8-5 A disto-angularly impacted third molar. Note the limited space between it and the second molar tooth and the hook at the apex of the third molar.

removed. When caries is found, it is also important to check the distal aspect of the lower second molar for caries. In many cases, this may be more advanced in the second molar, particularly with mesioangular and horizontal impactions.

Bulbosity of the crown occasionally adds to the difficulty in removing third molars by aggravating the degree of impaction.

The roots

Number

Although most third molars have either one or two roots, the number is variable and there may be as many as four roots. In Fig 8-6, there are three large roots, the mesial root exhibiting hypercementosis. When the roots are large, they are easily identifiable. However, additional roots can be difficult to see, particularly when fine and spindly. In identifying individual roots, it is helpful to trace the outline of the periodontal ligament space. An indistinct apex can mean that two root apices are superimposed upon each other.

Root curvature

Straight roots, or those that are gently curved in a distal direction and follow the path of removal of the tooth, are regarded as favourable. Roots curved in a mesial direction or hooked roots are unfavourable and such teeth may require sectioning in order to deliver the root without fracture. It is important to note whether the individual roots have conflicting paths of with-

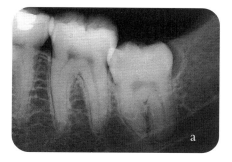
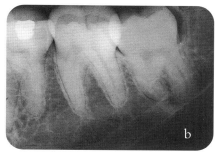

Fig 8-15 Vertical parallax radiographs of the same third molar showing the canal positioned differently on each film. The direction of change of position indicates that the canal lies buccal to the third molar roots. Fig 8-15a was taken with a 5° caudal (downward) tube angle and Fig 8-15b with a 10° cranial (upward) tube angulation. The cortices of the mandibular canal are positioned more apically in Fig 8-15a than in Fig 8-15b, confirming that it lies in a different plane from the roots and thus not grooving the roots.

Bone level

In order to determine the amount of bone covering the crown of an incompletely erupted lower third molar it is necessary to trace the level of the alveolar crest. For the bone level to be accurately shown, the radiograph should be taken using the paralleling technique so that a true lateral view of the tooth is obtained.

Bone density

The degree of bone density can be ascertained by the size of the marrow spaces (Fig 8-17). As the bone density increases the marrow spaces become smaller and the bone more radiopaque. The bone density obscures the detail and clarity of the root.

Other teeth

It is important to look at the other teeth particularly those in the same sextant.

• Look for caries, especially in the second molar.
• Note the root shape of second molar tooth. A conical root is more easily loosened than when this tooth has two stout roots.
• Look for root resorption.

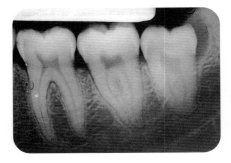

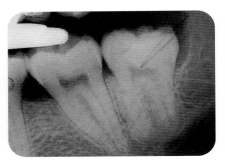

Fig 8-16 An enlarged distal follicular space, due to inflammatory hyperplasia. The tooth is vertically impacted and has a straight conical root. The enlarged follicular space has resulted in sufficient space to allow the tooth to be delivered without the need for distal bone removal. Note the sclerosing osteitis distal to the follicle space.

Fig 8-17 Increased bone density around a distoangularly impacted third molar. Note the small trabecular spaces and the apical hook on the third molar root.

Maxillary Canines

It is unusual for a maxillary canine to be congenitally absent. Thus, if one or both of these teeth fails to appear in the mouth at the expected time of eruption (Chapter 2) it is probably unerupted. A clinical examination must be undertaken before radiographing the patient. Look for local expansion of the buccal or palatal alveolus, which helps identify the presence and position of the unerupted tooth.

Radiographic Assessment of Maxillary Canines

Position
The factors that should be considered are: buccal/palatal displacement, angulation and depth in bone.

Bucco/palatal displacement
The buccopalatal location of an unerupted maxillary canine can be determined from parallax views (Chapter 1). These can be obtained with a tube shift by using two occlusal radiographs, or two periapical radiographs, or a combination of an occlusal and a periapical radiograph. Alternatively, a DPR can be used with an oblique occlusal film. An example of localisation of a buccal canine is shown in Fig 8-18 and of a palatal canine in Fig 8-19.

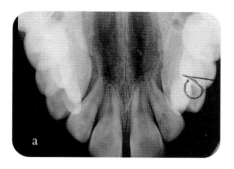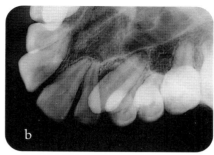

Fig 8-18 Upper anterior occlusal (a) and left oblique occlusal (b) radiographs showing an unerupted left maxillary canine. The canine is at the distal aspect of the root of the lateral incisor on the upper anterior occlusal (a). As the tube is move distally to take the upper oblique occlusal (b), the crown of the canine now adopts a more mesial position and overlies the distal half of the lateral incisor. Thus the unerupted maxillary canine has moved in the opposite direction to that of the tube shift, indicating that it is buccally displaced.

Angulation
Horizontally displaced canines tend to be more deeply placed than those that are mesio-angularly or vertically displaced.

Depth in bone
The depth of the tooth should be assessed by noting the proximity of the crown to the alveolar crest. Deeply placed maxillary canines will have their crowns close to the floor of the nose.

Crown and root form
Having determined the position of the canine, both the crown and the root should be individually assessed. The crown should be examined for caries and bulbosity. The canine root should be examines for:
• Length. Canines that are tilted may appear foreshortened. This may be compounded when using intra-oral views, particularly if the bisecting angle technique has been employed.
• Whether the apex is open or closed. A canine with an open apex still has eruptive potential.
• Curvature. Curved roots will add to the difficulty of removal.

Follicular size
The width of a normal follicular space is usually 2-4mm, but may exceed

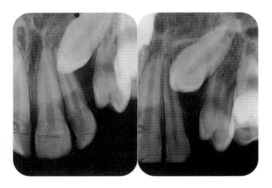

Fig 8-19 Two periapical radiographs, one centred on the upper incisor teeth and the other on the canine and first premolar region. The perspective change indicates that the canine is palatally displaced. Note that follicular space around the canine is enlarged.

this in maxillary canines. If the width is greater than 5mm it suggests the development of a dentigerous cyst (Fig 8-19).

Condition of other teeth
- Resorption of the lateral incisor.
- Root length of deciduous canine, if present.

Retained Roots

Retained roots are a common occurrence and most often result from an incomplete tooth extraction. The principles applied to the interpretation and assessment of lower third molars and maxillary canines can also be used to assess retained roots.

Buried tooth roots, when asymptomatic, may be discovered as an unexpected radiographic finding. To assess the root it is necessary to determine its:
- size
- closeness to the alveolar crest
- association with pathosis.

In many cases, particularly when the root is small and covered by bone, no abnormal radiological features are present. Such roots are best left on probation.

Roots may fracture during tooth extraction and in these cases a decision must be made whether to remove the fragment or leave it *in situ*. In Fig 8-20, the crown of the lower left second premolar has fractured during extraction, probably because of the bulbous root apex. If such a root is not removed and

Fig 8-20 Retained lower left second premolar root. There is no periapical radiographic change but the size of the fragment is such that if the root is left in situ it may subsequently become infected. The extraction of the root will require sufficient buccal bone removal to allow it to be delivered. If the root is to be removed, the position of the mental foramen should be assessed. In this case it lies at the distal aspect of the lower-left first premolar tooth.

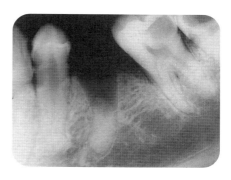

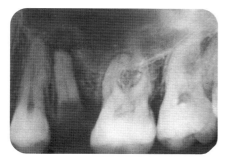

Fig 8-21 Grossly decayed upper first premolar tooth, with a periapical inflammatory lesion, which has resorbed part of the antral floor.

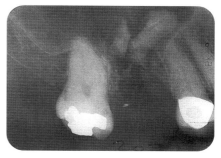

Fig 8-22 Roots displaced into the maxillary antrum during attempted elevation. The radiograph shows the low position of the antral floor in relation to the tooth socket.

the patient remains asymptomatic, the root should be radiographed in twelve months time to assess whether inflammatory change has taken place.

With upper teeth, potentially from canine to third molar, particular care should be exercised to assess the position of the antral floor. Consider, for example, the root shown in Fig 8-21. There is a periapical radiolucency affecting the grossly decayed upper left first premolar tooth that has resorbed the bone of the antral floor. This is shown by the discontinuity of its cortical outline. Thus, the root is vulnerable to being displaced into the antral cavity from the use of inappropriately applied extraction force. Fig 8-22 shows a case where the roots have been inadvertently been displaced in to the maxillary sinus.

Further Reading

Faculty of Dental Surgery. Current Clinical Parameters of Care: The Management of Patients with Third Molar Teeth. London: Royal College of Surgeons of England, 1977.

National Institute for Clinical Excellence. Guidance for the Removal of Wisdom Teeth. Technical Appraisal Guidance No.1. London: NICE, 2000.

Pedlar J, Frame JW. Oral and Maxillofacial Surgery: An Objective Based Textbook. Edinburgh: Churchill Livingstone, 2001.

Scottish Intercollegiate Guidelines Network. Management of Unerupted and Impacted Third Molar Teeth. A National Clinical Guideline. Edinburgh: SIGN, 2000.

Seward GR, Harris M, McGowan DA, Killey HC, Kay LW. An Outline of Oral Surgery. Parts 1 and 2. London: Reed Educational and Professional Publishing Ltd., 1988.

Whaites E. Developmental abnormalities. In: Whaites E. Essentials of Dental Radiography and Radiology. 3rd ed. Edinburgh: Churchill Livingstone, 2002: 271–283.

Chapter 9
Radiolucencies in the Jaws

Aim

The aim of this chapter is to provide a working knowledge of the more common types of radiolucencies and their differential diagnosis. Some uncommon radiolucencies have also been included to demonstrate the wide variety of lesions that may appear on dental radiographs.

Introduction

Faced with a radiolucency on a dental radiograph, the first questions to answer are:
- Is it anatomical?
- Is it artefactual?

The principal anatomical structures that are radiolucent (maxillary sinus, nasal cavity, foramina, etc.) have been described in Chapter 2. It is frequently variations in size or position of these normal structures that cause diagnostic problems.

As far as artefacts are concerned, a "radiolucent" (i.e. "dark") artefact can result from either overdevelopment (Fig 9-1) or localised exposure to x-rays or light (Fig 9-2).

If and when these causes of a radiolucency have been excluded, you must consider the pathological causes. Whilst inflammation remains the most common pathological reason for a radiolucency to appear in the jaw (see Chapter 5), there are inevitably many other causes that cannot be covered in their entirety in a book of this size. Table 9-1 provides an overview of this multiplicity of pathology, categorised using the surgical sieve as a template. You are referred to the further reading section at the end of this chapter should you wish to look into this subject in depth.

Choice of Radiographs

Periapical radiography is the "first-choice" examination of a small, localised

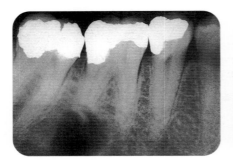 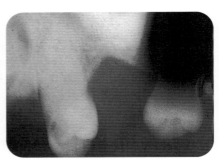

Fig 9-1 A "radiolucency" caused by a developer splash prior to processing. This patient almost underwent treatment for the "lesion".

Fig 9-2 A "radiolucency" produced by contamination by daylight from a perforation in the film packet.

lesion and provides optimal image detail. For larger pathosis, occlusal radiography can be useful in detailing not only the extent of the lesion but also the presence of bony expansion. Panoramic or oblique lateral radiography is needed only in those cases in which the pathosis is more extensive or multiple.

Assessing Radiolucencies in the Jaws

In practice, diagnosis of a radiolucency involves the analysis of certain radiological features, along with the details of the age, sex and racial group of the patient. Using these clinicoradiological features, the practitioner will be able, in the majority of patients, to arrive at a differential diagnosis or, occasionally, a definitive diagnosis. The principle radiographic signs to consider are listed below.

The Site of the Lesion

The probability that a lesion is odontogenic in origin is increased if it is found within alveolar bone and, in the mandible, if it lies above the mandibular canal.

The Shape of the Lesion

A round or ovoid appearance indicates a benign growth pattern such as is typically seen accompanying cysts and benign tumours. In larger cystic

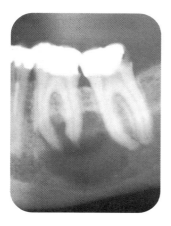

Fig 9-4 Radicular cyst associated with the heavily restored 36.

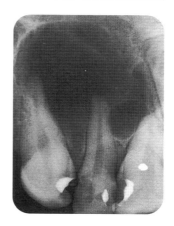

Fig 9-5 Large radicular cyst associated with a heavily restored 12. The margins are well defined with a thin cortical margin. The lamina dura of 12 is lost. Note that the small radiolucency mesial to 12 is the incisive foramen, not part of the lesion.

A residual cyst is a radicular cyst that remains in the jaw after the associated tooth has been extracted (Fig 9-6). The likeliest diagnosis for any pathological round/ovoid radiolucency with no relationship to a root or a crown in an adult is the residual cyst.

Dentigerous Cyst

The dentigerous cyst has a low incidence rate (< 10 per million per year-age standardised incidence rate) but represents the most common cyst in the jaws after the radicular cyst.

Clinical features

The lesion occurs most commonly in young adults. A clinical examination usually reveals reveal a missing tooth or a swelling in the jaw but the lesion is usually asymptomatic unless infected.

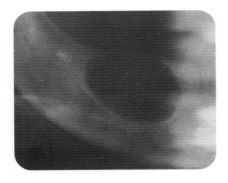

Fig 9-6 Residual cyst in an edentulous mandible. The ovoid, well-defined margin is the reassuringly benign feature.

Radiological signs

The most commonly affected tooth is the mandibular third molar followed by the maxillary canine. Supernumerary teeth and odontomes may also show cystic change. The normal follicular space measures 2-4 mm and, in the absence of robust scientific evidence to the contrary, a pragmatic approach would be to view follicular enlargement > 5mm as suspicious of cyst formation. A dentigerous cyst exhibits a well-defined symmetrical unilocular radiolucency associated with the crown of an unerupted tooth *(central type)*. A corticated margin delineates the periphery of the lesion and extends to the cementoenamel junction (Fig 9-7). Growth may lead to marked tooth displacement (Fig 9-8). As the cyst develops, it may envelop the tooth *(circumferential type)* or enlarge unilaterally (*lateral type* Fig 9-9) into an area offering less resistance to growth (i.e. the ascending ramus).

Expansion does occur but commonly affects only the buccal plate. Very occasionally multilocularity has been seen in large dentigerous cysts.

An eruption cyst is the alternative name for a dentigerous cyst when it is localised purely to soft tissue. The only radiological sign will be a soft tissue mass. A paradental cyst is the name given to a lesion that typically arises on the buccal surface of an impacted molar and involves the furcation; whether this is inflammatory in aetiology or developmental is not entirely clear.

Lateral Periodontal Cyst

This lesion is more unusual and the diagnosis is reserved for those lesions in a lateral periodontal position for which an inflammatory cause or a keratocyst has been excluded both clinically and histopathologically.

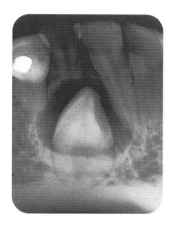

Fig 9-7 Dentigerous cyst (central type) associated with an unerupted 43.

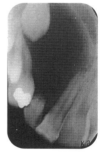

Fig 9-8 Large dentigerous cyst of an ectopic 13, causing displacement of 12.

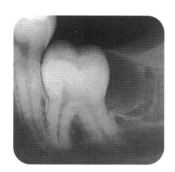

Fig 9-9. Dentigerous cyst (lateral type) on 38.

Clinical features

The patient is usually asymptomatic unless the lesion becomes infected. The condition is seen more commonly in males. Most cases occur between the fifth and sixth decades and the associated tooth is vital unless otherwise affected. Slight buccal swelling has been reported in a small proportion of patients.

Radiological signs

In two-thirds of cases, the lesion is limited to the mandibular premolar/canine/incisor region with the remainder occurring in the maxillary lateral/canine region. The lesion presents as an oval or round unilocu-

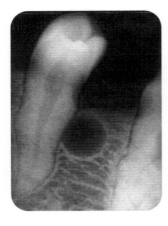

Fig 9-10 Lateral periodontal cyst on 45. The tooth has no other pathosis.

lar radiolucency (< 1cm) and with a well-defined and corticated margin. It is positioned midway between the cervical and apical region of the root (Fig 9-10) and resorption of the adjacent lamina dura may be evident.

Keratocyst

The keratocyst is a developmental odontogenic cyst, making up about one-tenth of all jaw cysts, with an incidence rate of less than 5 per million per year in white populations (much less in black people).

Clinical features
The cyst is slightly more common in males and found most frequently during the second and third decades. The posterior mandible is most commonly affected. The patient is usually asymptomatic as bone expansion is an uncommon finding with the lesion preferring to extend along the medullary cavity. The keratocyst can recur following surgical treatment and requires extended radiographic follow-up.

Radiological signs
The keratocyst presents as either a round or ovoid unilocular or, in the case of larger lesions, a multilocular radiolucency. The margins of lesions are either smooth or scalloped (Fig 9-11). It has been suggested that the characteristic scalloped or pseudoloculated appearance is a result of differential growth activity within the cyst lining. Both unilocular and multilocular types of keratocyst display a well-corticated margin. Enlarging keratocysts may

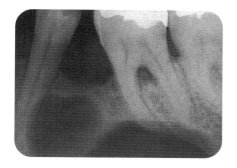 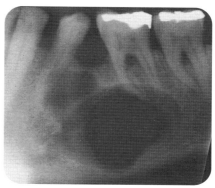

Fig 9-11a,b Keratocyst in the left mandible of a 50-year-old man on periapical (a) and panoramic (b) views. Note the scalloped sclerotic margins that are classic features of this lesion.

deflect roots and unerupted teeth but root resorption is rarely seen. Keratocysts are a feature of Gorlin-Goltz syndrome (basal cell naevus syndrome), an inherited condition. Clinical features of this condition include cutaneous abnormalities (basal cell carcinomas, palmar and/or plantar pits) and osseous abnormalities that include multiple jaw cysts.

Nasopalatine Cyst

The nasopalatine cyst is a non-odontogenic cyst and has an incidence rate similar to that of the keratocyst.

Clinical features

The age distribution is broad although the majority of cysts occur during the fourth, fifth and sixth decades. Small nasopalatine cysts are usually asymptomatic or the patient may complain of a salty discharge. Pain and altered sensation are often reported accompanying larger lesions, as is swelling in the anterior region of the palate and/or the labial alveolar ridge. Vitality tests are important to distinguish the lesion from a radicular cyst.

Radiological signs

The nasopalatine cyst is located in the midline of the anterior palate (Fig 9-12) and appears as a well-defined round or ovoid radiolucency with a corticated margin (unless infected). The lesion may present rarely as a bi-lobular or heart-shaped radiolucency due to the simultaneous development of bilateral cysts. The presence of an intact lamina dura surrounding the maxillary

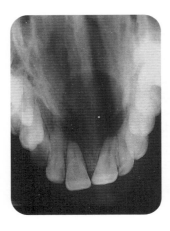

Fig 9-12 Nasopalatine cyst on an occlusal radiograph. This lesion is classical in its symmetry; 21 is displaced.

central incisors is useful in distinguishing it from a radicular cyst, but as the lesion enlarges lamina dura can be eroded. The distinction between a small cyst and a normal incisive foramen is usually made on size. The incisive foramen is typically about 6 mm in width but may be as much as 10 mm anteroposteriorly (see Chapter 2). In addition, a normal incisive fossa is sharply delineated only at its lateral margin, whereas all margins of a nasopalatine cyst are well defined.

Solitary Bone Cyst

This rare lesion (incidence rate about 1 per million per year) is also known as a haemorrhagic, simple or traumatic bone cyst. The aetiology and pathogenesis of the condition remain unknown.

Clinical features

The solitary bone cyst occurs most frequently in children. However, multiple cysts have been reported in older individuals with cemento-osseous lesions (see Chapter 10). The majority of patients are asymptomatic. The teeth associated with the solitary bone cyst are vital (unless otherwise affected).

Radiological signs

The majority of lesions are found in the premolar/molar region of the mandible (Fig 9-13). The margins are generally either oval or scalloped superiorly, the latter producing a pseudolocular appearance. In the superior aspect of the lesion the margins may be seen arching upwards between the roots of

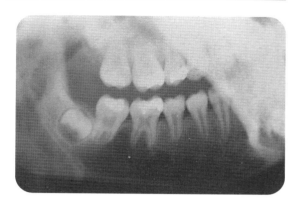

Fig 9-13 Solitary bone cyst in the right molar region. The lesion has grown between the roots of the molars without displacing or resorbing them.

the teeth. Expansion is infrequent.

Ameloblastoma

Ameloblastoma is a benign but locally aggressive neoplasm of odontogenic epithelium. It is rare representing 1% of all oral tumours.

Clinical features

Ameloblastomas are found slightly more commonly in males and between the ages of 20 and 50. The lesion exhibits relatively slow growth and presents as a painless swelling accompanied by tooth displacement and mobility. The ameloblastoma can recur following surgical treatment.

Radiological signs

Most ameloblastomas (80%) are found in the posterior regions of the mandible. The ameloblastoma usually has a well-defined corticated margin that is either smooth or scalloped. It can be either unilocular or multilocular (Fig 9-14). Ameloblastomas cause expansion, tooth displacement, thinning of the cortical plate and "knife-edge" resorption of root apices. Both buccal and lingual expansion is evident accompanying larger lesions. Root resorption is a common feature.

Metastatic Deposits

The commonest intra-bony malignancies in the jaws are metastatic carcinomas. Radiolucent metastatic deposits develop from primary lesions such as breast, lung, kidney, thyroid, colon, skin, bladder, testes and ovary. Of these, breast, lung, kidney and colon are the most common primary tumours

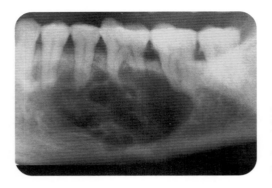

Fig 9-14 Ameloblastoma of the left mandible in a 45-year-old man (panoramic view). Note the multilocular appearance and the root resorption of 35 and 36.

that metastasise to the jaws, with the posterior mandible, especially the third molar region, being the most common site (> 80%).

Clinical features

The average age of patients presenting with metastatic disease is 55. Pain is the most frequent symptom followed by swelling, paraesthesia, loosening of teeth and occasionally pathological fracture.

Radiological signs

Metastases can present in several ways. In the multifocal type of metastatic disease, there are several non-corticated but well delineated radiolucencies in the posterior mandible separated by normal bone. The alternative pattern is of multiple small lytic areas that have a "moth-eaten" /infiltrative pattern separated by minimal areas of normal bone (Fig 9-15). As the lesions expand these isolated areas will coalesce forming a larger ill-defined radiolucency. There is often loss of the lamina dura of adjacent teeth and "floating" teeth

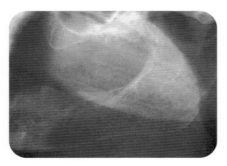

Fig 9-15 Metastatic carcinoma in the mandible of a 70-year-old woman. There is a diffuse radiolucency of the entire body of mandible and, most importantly, extreme resorption of the lower border cortex. This patient presented after feeling her jaw "crack". Subsequent films demonstrated a subtle pathological fracture through the jaw.

may also be seen. In advanced cases, bone loss may be extensive involving the cortical plates.

Surgical (Fibrous Healing) Defect

This is a complication following a difficult or surgical extraction or apicectomy. It can also been seen as a post-operative feature following extensive jaw surgery. In such cases, loss of the periosteum leads to repair by fibrous intention. The defect is, of course, asymptomatic.

Radiological signs

Lesions can occur anywhere in the jaws but the maxillary anterior and premolar regions are common. It presents as an extremely radiolucent lesion of variable shape with a well-defined, "punched out" margin (Fig 9-16).

Giant Cell Granuloma

The giant cell granuloma is considered as a reactive lesion, accounting for 7% of benign jaw lesions.

Clinical features

The lesion commonly affects young people with almost two-thirds of cases occurring in individuals below 30 years of age, although the range is wide. Females are affected more commonly. Most patients present with a painless, swelling in the anterior mandible or maxilla that occurs rapidly and displaces teeth.

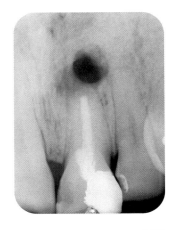

Fig 9-16 Surgical (fibrous healing) defect on 21. This tooth had undergone apicectomy in the past for a small cyst.

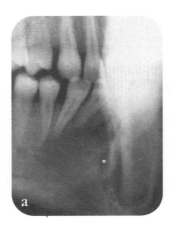
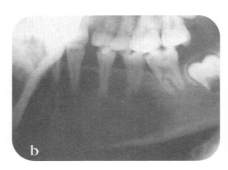

Fig 9-17a,b Right (a) and left (b) oblique lateral radiographs of the mandible showing a patient with an extensive giant cell granuloma centred upon the mandibular midline. The margins are not so well defined, reflecting a rapid growth. There is some evidence of multilocularity on the left side.

Radiological signs

The giant cell granuloma occurs in the mandible in two-thirds of cases. Although lesions do occur in the posterior aspects of the jaw, the majority of lesions develop anterior to the first permanent molar with almost a fifth crossing the mid-line. The smaller lesion (< 2cm) is a radiolucency with a well-defined margin. The larger lesion will show an irregular shape with a sclerotic periphery exhibiting a scalloped or undulating appearance. Larger lesions (Fig 9-17) can exhibit pronounced bucco-lingual expansion and multilocularity with straight, thin, wispy septae projecting at right angles from the periphery. It can cause displacement of unerupted teeth and the lamina dura of adjacent teeth is often missing. Aggressive lesions can cause root resorption and perforation of the expanded cortex.

Hyperparathyroidism

Primary hyperparathyroidism results from an excessive secretion of parathyroid hormone (PTH) resulting, most commonly, from an adenoma of a gland (90%) or hyperplasia of all four glands (5%). Secondary and tertiary causes of hyperparathyroidism may also occur.

Clinical features

Middle-aged women are more commonly affected by primary hyper-

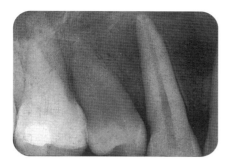 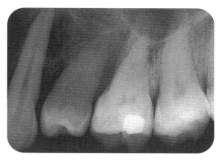

Fig 9-18 Hyperparathyroidism. Both films demonstrate a generalised loss of lamina dura and a featureless trabecular pattern of the bone.

parathyroidism. The clinical picture has been described as "bones, stones, abdominal groans and psychic moans with fatigue overtones", reflecting the presence of generalised demineralisation of bone, renal calculi, peptic ulcers and psychiatric problems. Most cases are identified by haematology rather than by radiology.

Radiological signs

There is a generalised osteopaenia (loss of bone density) within the jaws and a thinning of cortices. The normal trabecular pattern is altered with a fine granular appearance. The lamina dura of the teeth is lost (Fig 9-18) either generally or locally. Localised bone lesions also occur within the jaws as the disease progresses. These are referred to as "brown tumours". They are often multiple.

Further Reading

Shear M. Cysts of the Oral Regions. 3rd ed. Bristol: Wright, 1992.

Whaites E. Differential Diagnosis of Radiolucent Lesions of the Jaws. In: Whaites E. Essentials of Dental Radiography and Radiology. 3rd ed. Edinburgh: Churchill Livingstone, 2002: 291–316.

White SC, Pharoah MJ. Cysts of the jaws. In: White SC, Pharoah MJ (Eds.) Oral Radiology. Principles and Interpretation. 4th ed. St Louis: Mosby, 2000.

Wood NK, Goaz PW. Differential Diagnosis of Oral and Maxillofacial Lesions. 5th ed. St Louis: Mosby, 1997: 238–413.

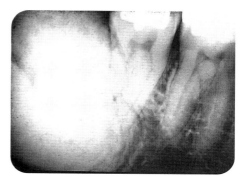

Fig 10-4 A large complex odontome in 48 region. Like the compound variety, the complex odontome has a thin radiolucent capsule. The high radiopacity reflects the enamel content.

Clinical features

The likeliest presenting feature is failure of eruption of a tooth or teeth. The most common site is the molar region of the mandible.

Radiological signs

The complex odontome is generally larger than the compound type. It is a densely radiopaque mass without any regular internal structure (Fig 10-4). A radiolucent capsule should be discernible.

Sclerosing osteitis

This inflammatory reaction within bone, typically associated with dental disease, is described in Chapter 5.

Socket sequestrum

Extraction of a tooth may leave fragments of socket wall that are devitalised and that act as sequestra.

Clinical features

It is likely that small fragments of bone are very common and cause no problems. You are most likely to identify one when a patient returns in pain after an extraction. There is likely to be obvious inflammation, debris and pus in the socket and the sequestrum may be visible, or palpable using a probe.

Radiological signs

The sequestrum will be visible as an irregular radiopaque mass overlying the socket, with a line of demarcation separating it from normal bone (Fig 10-5).

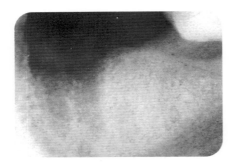

Fig 10-5 Socket sequestrum. This patient had undergone extraction of 36 two weeks previously, but had suffered "infection" in the socket. The sequestrum appears as the irregular radiopacity at the top of the socket, with a thin demarcating line between it and the underlying bone.

Osteomyelitis

See Chapter 5.

Osteosclerosis

Also known as "idiopathic osteosclerosis" or "dense bone island". This condition commonly causes diagnostic problems for dentists.

Clinical features

There are no clinical signs or symptoms. The abnormality is a chance radiographic finding.

Radiological signs

Usually in the mandibular premolar or molar regions, it appears as a focal area of increased bone density. The shape is irregular and variable, but the margins are sharp. Typically it is found around the root or roots of lower posterior teeth (Fig 10-6). In some cases, the condition is not found against a tooth root, but may be positioned either between the roots or in the basal bone (Fig 10-7). It has been postulated that the cause for some of these dense bone islands is low-grade irritation from a retained deciduous tooth root remnant. Such an example is shown in Fig 10-8, where there is a central area of increased radiodensity that could represent a submerged distal root apex of a primary second molar. If this is the explanation for this condition, the origin is an inflammatory one, but in most cases it is difficult to prove as the density is such that a root fragment is obscured.

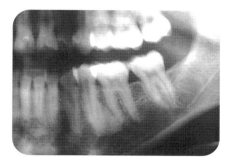

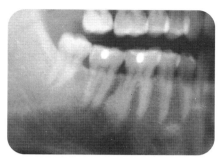

Fig 10-6 Osteosclerosis in the mandibular left second premolar region. Here there is an irregularly shaped radiopacity which appears to involve the distal aspect of the lower second premolar, and which extends to the mesial root of the lower first molar.

Fig 10-7 Two areas of osteosclerosis, lying between the premolar apices and around the distal root of the lower-right first molar. As there is a filling in 46, this lesion could be due to sclerosing osteitis. The filling, however, appears small so the diagnosis seems most probably osteosclerosis.

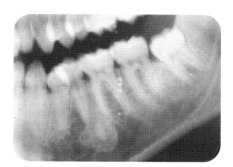

Fig 10-8 Osteosclerosis, possibly containing a primary root fragment.

Fibro-Cemento-Osseous Lesions

This refers to a group of conditions in which bone is replaced by fibrous tissue that, in turn, then undergoes mineralisation by cementum or bone. Histologically, it can be difficult to distinguish bone from cementum and hence cementum and osseous-containing conditions are considered together. Their radiographic appearance depends on the relative amounts of fibrous and calcified tissues.

The group consists of:
• periapical cemental dysplasia
• florid cemento-osseous dysplasia

- cemento-ossifying fibroma
- benign cementoblastoma.

The last is very rare. The first two are, in contrast, relatively frequent and important to the dentist. As such we will concentrate solely upon these "cemento-osseous dysplasias".

Clinical features
Both periapical cemental dysplasia and florid cemento-osseous dysplasia are found mainly in middle-aged women, particularly Afrocaribbean and Asian women. They are asymptomatic and so discovered as an incidental radiographic finding. Several lesions develop especially around lower incisors and first molars roots, although any tooth may be involved. The affected teeth maintain their vitality. As the condition is self-limiting, it requires monitoring rather than surgical intervention. The "florid" form is characterised by larger multi-quadrant lesions.

Radiological features
This depends on the stage of development. Initially the fibrous tissue component predominates resulting in a periapical radiolucency with a well-defined margin (Fig 10-9). During this phase, it resembles a periapical inflammatory lesion (see Chapter 5). As the lesion matures, cementum or bone is deposited, so that it now appears as a mixed-density lesion. These deposits of cementum are surrounded by a zone of radiolucency. In the third or final stage when further mineralisation has taken place, the lesion becomes almost entirely radiopaque, except for a thin peripheral radiolucent capsular space (Fig 10-10). An example of the florid form is shown in Fig 10-11. Occasionally, solitary bone cysts (see Chapter 9) may develop in patients with florid cemento-osseous dysplasia.

Fibrous Dysplasia

In this condition, normal cancellous bone is replaced by fibrous tissue that subsequently undergoes mineralisation to varying degrees. The condition may affect one bone (monostotic) or there may be more than one bony lesion (polyostotic) and when associated with endocrine and skin pigmentation is known as the McCune-Albright syndrome. The bones commonly affected are the ribs, femur and tibia and the jaws.

Clinical features
This is a condition that occurs during childhood as a bony swelling and which

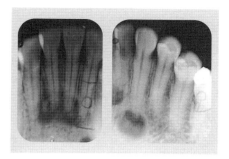
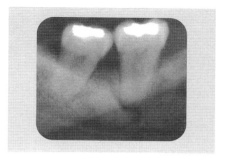

Fig 10-9 Early and intermediate periapical cemental dysplasia. There are periapical radiolucencies involving both lower central incisors and 32, along with a separate lesion on 33.

Fig 10-10 Late-stage periapical cemental dysplasia. There is a large radiopaque mass with a thin radiolucent margin. Note the radiopacity difference between this lesion and the complex odontome in Fig 10-4.

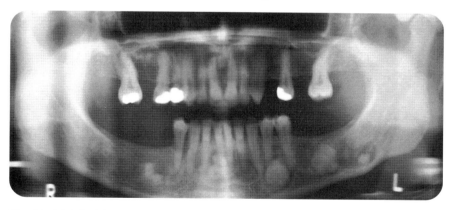

Fig 10-11 Florid osseous dysplasia. There are multiple radiopaque masses in the mandible.

usually arrests around the time of puberty. There is no gender predilection except in the McCune-Albright syndrome, which mainly affects females. Jaw lesions tend to be solitary and unilateral and occur more commonly in the maxilla than mandible. They are usually painless.

Radiological signs
The lesion may be largely radiolucent, but more often is seen as a radiopacity. Typically, the bone has an altered trabecular pattern, which is seen as a

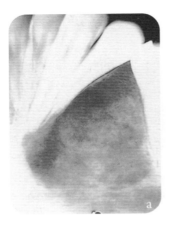 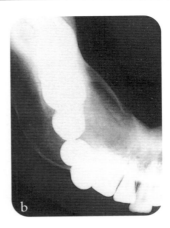

Fig 10-12 Periapical (a) and lower true occlusal (b) views of a mainly radiolucent fibrous dysplasia, in the lower-left premolar region. It is well defined and contains evidence of mineralisation. There is displacement of the tooth roots. The occlusal radiograph (b) shows expansion and thinning of the buccal and lingual cortical plates, which remain intact.

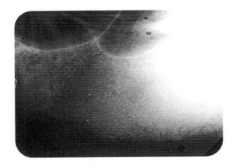

Fig 10-13 Orange peel effect typically associated with fibrous dysplasia, in the left maxilla. This manifestation is more likely to be seen as the lesion becomes denser with age. The stippled appearance is more likely to be visible on intra-oral radiographs than extra-oral films due to its better resolution.

"ground glass" or "stippled" appearance. Except in the radiolucent type the margins are usually indistinct so that the lesion tends to merge with the normal surrounding bone. Large lesions will expand, rather than perforate the cortical plates, so that in the maxilla, for example, the antral floor may be raised but remain intact. Fibrous dysplasia may displace the teeth or interfere with normal eruption. Examples of the condition are shown in Figs 10-12a,b and 10-13.

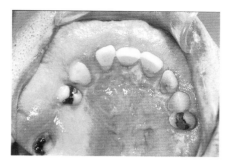

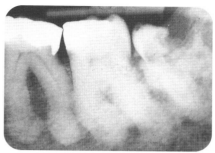

Fig 10-14 Clinical photograph of a patient with Paget's disease affecting the maxilla. The alveolar bone is grossly expanded buccally.

Fig 10-15 Paget's disease of the mandible. The teeth show hypercementosis and have lost lamina dura. The trabecular pattern is abnormal, with a horizontal pattern.

Paget's Disease of Bone

This is a condition where the normal processes of bone turnover, bone resorption and deposition become uncoordinated. It can affect several bones including the spine, long bones, skull and jaws. However, it is important to recognise that a patient may have the disease without jaw involvement.

Clinical features

Paget's disease mainly affects the middle aged or elderly. Sometimes the patient will complain of bone pain and when skull foramina are compressed the patient may have neurological pain, deafness or blindness. It may affect the maxilla or mandible and when it does so it causes bilateral expansion as it involves the whole jaw. The clinical appearance is of an expanded alveolus (Fig 10-14). The teeth become separated as the jaw enlarges. Alternatively, the patient may complain that they are unable to insert their dentures.

Radiological signs

The bone progresses through an osteolytic and osteoblastic phase, which usually occur simultaneously, but with the osteblastic phase being ultimately more dominant. Thus, the radiographic appearance is that of an increased radiopacity of the jaws. The bone tends to become more granular in appearance and the lamina dura is obscured or difficult to identify (Fig 10-15). Here the bony trabeculae, particularly in the posterior part of the body of the mandible, may show linear striations. In addition, the teeth show hypercementosis (Fig 10-15). A more classical appearance is that of granular- looking

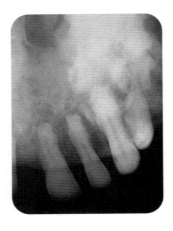

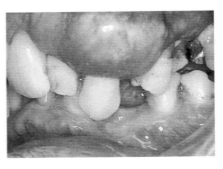

Fig 10-17 Clinical photograph of an osteoma of the maxilla. It had shown slow but continued growth, with displacement of the upper canine, which was now traumatising the mucosa of the mandible.

Fig 10-16 Paget's disease of the maxilla on an occlusal radiograph showing hypercementosis, expansion of the alveolus and patchy radiopacity.

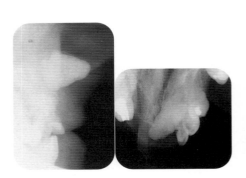

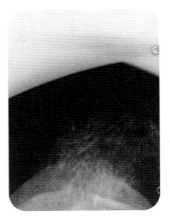

Fig 10-18 True lateral and periapical radiographs showing a compact osteoma.

Fig 10-19 A large cancellous osteoma shown on an occlusal view of the anterior aspect of the mandible.

bone containing scattered islands of dense or fluffy-looking bone, particularly in the region of the tooth apices (Fig 10-16).

Osteoma

There is some confusion whether osteomas are benign tumours of bone or